Foundations for Practice in Occupational Therapy

Rosemary Hagedorn DipCOT DipTCDHEd MSc(AOT) FCOT
Freelance author and lecturer, Arundel, UK

THIRD EDITION

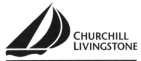
CHURCHILL
LIVINGSTONE

EDINBURGH LONDON NEW YORK PHILADELPHIA ST LOUIS SYDNEY TORONTO 2001

CHURCHILL LIVINGSTONE
An imprint of Harcourt Publishers Limited

First edition 1992
Second edition 1997
Third edition 2001

ISBN 0 443 06470 9

British Library Cataloguing in Publication Data
A catalogue record for this book is available from the British Library

Library of Congress Cataloging in Publication Data
A catalog record for this book is available from the Library of Congress

Note
Medical knowledge is constantly changing. As new information becomes available, changes in treatment, procedures, equipment and the use of drugs become necessary. The author and the publishers have taken care to ensure that the information given in this text is accurate and up to date. However, readers are strongly advised to confirm that the information, especially with regard to drug usage, complies with the latest legislation and standards of practice.

The
publisher's
policy is to use
**paper manufactured
from sustainable forests**

Printed in China

Foundations for Practice in Occupational Therapy

For Churchill Livingstone:

Editorial Director: Mary Law
Project Manager: Gail Murray
Project Development Manager: Dinah Thom
Designer: George Ajayi

Contents

Preface

ABOUT THIS BOOK

This book evolved out of a simple student handbook on 'models' written around 1989, as an aid to teaching what seemed at the time an arcane topic.

The first edition was published in 1992. I am somewhat astonished, eight years later, to find myself engaged in the production of a third edition.

The aim of the book is to provide a guide to, and summary of, frames of reference and models of practice. In this new edition I have completely revised the introductory section and included a section on person-environment-occupational performance models. I have also made a particular effort to update references and reading lists.

Although some of the mystery has diminished, the topic remains challenging. As before, the book will not tell you 'what to think and what to do'; it will offer you guidance on 'how to think' and a range of theoretical structures to guide that process. I hope it proves as useful as the previous editions.

ABOUT MYSELF

Every author has a past. The past colours perceptions and produces a personal world furnished with beliefs, values and prejudices from which the author cannot escape, even if she tries. Experience, however rich, is always partial; there are bound to be gaps. I believe it is important for you to understand that, and to read this book with a critical and questioning attitude.

To that end it may be useful for you to know a little about my professional background. I qualified as an occupational therapist in 1965 and worked mainly with adults or older people who had physical disabilities or injuries. Later, as a district occupational therapist, I managed a range of services including those for clients with learning disabilities and people with mental health disorders. In 1986 I made a sideways jump into education as Head of the Crawley Occupational Therapy School.

On leaving Crawley College I took some time out for personal development via an MSc in Advanced Occupational Therapy, and returned to part-time clinical practice to touch base with the realities of occupational therapy 'at the sharp end', including involvement in pain management and research into falls in older people.

Along the route of the past ten years of that journey I have written books, and by the act of immersion in theory (following the dictum that 'by doing we become') I find myself somehow transmuted into 'a theorist'. I have now retired from practice and am busy 'doing and becoming' in other personal occupations.

WHAT NEXT?

Over the past decade occupational therapy has achieved a firm theoretical foundation. In particular, the unique cluster of perceptions concerning occupation and its central importance in human life has been made explicit.

We do not need more theory; we need time to consolidate, refine and evaluate what we have. Above all, we now need to explore the relevance of theory to practice, and to test and document the effectiveness of our models and techniques where it really matters, not in academic discussion but in our daily contacts with our clients.

Development of theory and philosophy, while necessary, can be an inward-looking, and therefore isolating, process. We claim to be client-centred. Being client-centred means that we need to listen. Perhaps the time has come to involve our clients in the discussion of our concepts and values, and in testing their practical application.

Occupational therapy has had a long childhood and an over-extended period of defensive and insecure adolescence. Having attained adulthood (if not yet, perhaps, maturity) we face interesting challenges in externalizing and promoting our practice in a positive and open dialogue with our employers and our clients.

As I move away from the profession which has consumed my energy and enthusiasm for thirty-five years, I look forward to seeing how the next generation of therapists will take this important field of practice into the twenty-first century.

Arundel 2000   Rosemary Hagedorn

An introduction to philosophy, principles and practice

1

INTRODUCTION

THE PURPOSE OF THIS BOOK

This is a book about ideas. It deals with the 'whys' and 'whats' of occupational therapy (OT) rather than the 'hows'. For the latter you will need to refer to other sources which are listed in the references.

The book is intended for use as a basic text for students who need to understand the theoretical foundations for practice. It should also be helpful to more experienced therapists who wish to take an analytical approach to their work or to extend or update their theoretical vocabulary and concepts. It may perhaps assist non-therapists to achieve a better understanding of the scope and basis of occupational therapy.

There are many frames of reference and theoretical models to guide the practice of occupational therapy. Getting to grips with the concepts and language can be daunting and bewildering. Where do all these conceptual constructs come from? Why are they useful? Which one is appropriate in which situation? How does theory relate to what the therapist actually does with the patient or client? What does all the jargon mean?

It is hoped that in reading this book you will be guided towards some of the answers. The material is presented at introductory level. Models and frames of reference are summarized and it is necessary to do additional reading if you intend to put a particular model into practice. References and reading lists are provided.

THE CONTENTS OF THIS BOOK

The text is arranged in four sections.

Section 1 provides an introduction to the philosophy, principles and practice of OT. Some key concepts concerning the philosophical and theoretical basis of the profession are defined and summarized. The external and internal factors which have contributed to development of OT theory are explored. Finally this section describes the processes of occupational therapy and makes links between theory and practice through the mechanisms of clinical reasoning.

Section 2 describes frames of reference derived from sources external to occupational therapy and those modified by therapists for use in OT.

Section 3 describes the process of change affecting the individual which may be used by the therapist to assist the client to achieve personal goals.

Section 4 deals with person-environment-occupational performance models which have been developed by occupational therapists specifically for use within occupational therapy.

ADVICE TO READERS

You are invited to take a critical approach to the material in this book. Ideas are not to be accepted at face value just because someone has written them down. In order to understand theory you will need to engage actively with the material. You can do this through discussion, writing and by exploring case studies and analysing practice. I have occasionally included a question box to stimulate these exercises.

Theory can be challenging and difficult to grasp when you encounter it for the first time. You do need to persevere past the initial onset of intellectual overload, semantic confusion and aching brain! Do not attempt to deal with too much information at once – to do so will result in a bad attack of mental 'indigestion'.

UNDERSTANDING OCCUPATIONAL THERAPY

Occupational therapy is a complex profession. It has a broad knowledge base, derived from both medical and social sciences. Practice merges managerial, remedial, technical and creative skills with the specialized processes of occupational therapy. Therapists work with all age groups and assist with a wide range of medical, social and environmental problems.

Definitions

There are many definitions of occupational therapy; only a few of the more widely accepted ones will be given here.

In 1989 the World Federation of Occupational Therapists defined occupational therapy as follows:

Occupational therapy is the treatment of physical and psychiatric conditions through specific activities to help people to reach their maximum level of function and independence.

The College of Occupational Therapists (UK) issued a position statement in 1994 on Core Skills and the Conceptual Foundation for Practice which stated that:

The occupational therapist assesses the physical, psychological and social functions of the individual, identifies areas of dysfunction and involves the individual in a structured programme of activity to overcome disability. The activities selected will relate to the consumer's personal, social, cultural and economic needs and will reflect the evironmental factors which govern his life.

The Committee of Occupational Therapists for the European Community (COTEC) provides a brief definition:

Occupational therapists assess and treat people using purposeful activity to prevent disability and develop independent function.

Whilst these definitions have the virtue of brevity they fail to convey the full scope of current OT practice. There are many other definitions and descriptions, mostly lengthy, and all subject to criticism. It is an interesting exercise to attempt to write one's own definition; it provides a lesson in the problems of constructing a satisfactory, informative summary of something as multifaceted as occupational therapy.

It is important that therapists are familiar with the available definitions and that each practitioner has a full understanding of the principles, purposes and scope of the profession, and is able to convey this to others.

THE SCOPE OF OT

General and specialized areas of practice

In Britain the majority of occupational therapists work either within the National Health Service in hospitals and clinics or are employed by Social Services to work in the community.

The professional training for occupational therapy may follow a variety of routes, both full-time and part-time, and includes a specified amount of clinical experience. Training typically involves a degree course, although postgraduate diploma courses are also available. State registration is a prerequisite for work in most areas.

Specialisms such as learning disabilities, paediatrics, neurology, hand rehabilitation, and forensic psychiatry require additional training and experience.

A minority of occupational therapists are employed by other organizations, including the private health care sector, and charities. Some experienced therapists are in private practice where they act as consultants or specialize in medico-legal work. With this breadth of work it may readily be appreciated that occupational therapists need to draw on many sources of knowledge concerning people, their occupations and their environments, and that no single theory or approach would be likely to suffice.

THE PRINCIPAL CONCERNS OF OT

During the last decade of the 20th century there was an active debate within the profession about the fundamental principles of occupational therapy and the way in which these should be expressed. The debate is ongoing, but some consensus is emerging.

Occupational therapy:

- Is concerned with the key elements of occupational performance: the individual and the roles, occupations, and relationships which that person has in the environment which he or she inhabits.
- Aims to enable and empower people to be competent and confident performers in their daily lives, and thereby to enhance well-being and minimize the effects of dysfunction or environmental barriers.

Occupational therapists:

- Encourage individuals to engage actively in the processes of therapy and to become partners with the therapist in designing and directing this process.
- Use activities and tasks creatively and therapeutically to achieve goals which are meaningful to the person and relevant to his daily life.

These principles are informed by a set of humanistic values which emphasize the importance of personal experience, meanings and autonomous choices.

OCCUPATIONAL PERFORMANCE

Each person wants to be an effective actor in the world, and to remain healthy and happy. To achieve these goals a person needs a degree of personal competence in a range of culturally accepted, useful and meaningful occupations, activities and tasks. *Occupational performance* is the act of engagement in such occupations and daily activities.

Competence and dysfunction

Occupational therapists believe that competent occupational performance depends on a complex interaction between the individual, his environment, and the things he does. Well-being is directly related to the quality of this interaction.

When a person is performing competently he or she is usually able to meet the demands of each task, to respond adaptively to the demands of each environment, and to use the skills and knowledge he or she has learnt in order to act, interact and react appropriately in all the everyday situations which are encountered.

The opposite to occupational competence is *occupational dysfunction*. This is a temporary or chronic inability to engage in the roles, relationships and occupations expected of a person of comparable age and sex within a particular culture. Occupational dysfunction becomes apparent when a person is unable to do the ordinary everyday things he wants or needs to do.

The reasons for dysfunction are very variable and range from the simple to the extremely complex. They include factors which come from the external world and also factors which come from within the individual.

In a simple case the individual may, for example, have damage due to a physical injury or illness. Reactions to physical damage are closely related to the demands of the roles and occupations of the person concerned; the same condition may have a very adverse affect on one person, and very little on another.

The OT perspective

The therapist needs to understand the nature of the client's occupations in relation to the health condition and its prognosis. Using an appropriate frame of reference, action can be taken to improve the patient's physical condition, and/or to reduce the impact on his or her ability to engage in activities. Theoretical frameworks for intervention of this kind are explained in Section 2.

Therapists are not, however, limited to consideration of the impact of health problems on an individual's life, important though these may be. Dysfunction is frequently associated with a failure to adapt to a set of circumstances which has overloaded the capacity of the individual to respond.

Most people become dysfunctional to some extent when faced with an unfamiliar or difficult situation or when confronted by a very stressful life event. Such dysfunction is usually transient and either resolves when the stress is removed, responds to minimal advice or assistance or disappears once the person has learned how to cope. This type of dysfunction may arise from external factors in the absence of any impairment or health condition.

The kind of complex occupational dysfunction which requires intervention from an occupational therapist is persistent, and often affects many aspects of the individual's life.

Occupational therapists use the processes of occupational therapy (see Chapter 4) and the processes of change (see Section 3) to assist the client to develop personal goals and work towards achieving them.

The social and physical environment can inhibit or enhance performance. In addition, the nature of the task and the circumstances of its performance also have an effect. Occupational therapists believe that alteration of these external factors can have crucial importance when seeking to restore competence.

One way of looking at dysfunction is to describe it as a lack of balance or 'fit' between the skills of the individual, the challenges of the environment and the difficulties of the task.

The individual may have lost skills or never have learnt them. He may have some negative emotional reaction connected with the task. The physical environment may be badly designed, too demanding or not demanding enough. The social environment may be too stressful or insufficiently supportive. The task may be too difficult or the tools inappropriate.

The role of the occupational therapist is to intervene to help the individual to balance these factors and regain competence.

The therapist may adapt the performance demand of the task, alter the environment in some way, teach the individual a new repertoire of skills or help him to re-establish ones he has lost. The theoretical basis of such intervention is explained in Section 4.

2

Theoretical foundation of OT: external influences

WHAT IS THEORY?

Theory is an over-used word with many meanings. We use it to mean the opposite of practice; we talk of theories when we mean speculative ideas or *hypotheses*; we may imply that someone's theory is 'just ideas' – not of much use.

In the context of models of practice a theory is 'an attempt to bind together in a systematic fashion the knowledge that one has of some particular aspect of the world or experience' (Honderich 1995).

A theory promotes understanding, and may predict occurrences under certain conditions or offer a logical argument or set of proofs to support what is being said. This is the traditional scientific view of theory. Theories of this type are 'weighted' in accordance with the quality and reliability of the evidence: research involving many controlled trials has the most credibility. Ideas which stem from descriptions or untested hypotheses have the least. A theory may stand until disproved and replaced by a new theory.

The nature of theory is, however, subject to dispute. Recent thinkers have challenged the traditional scientific view, seeing theories more as a set of possible, even alternative, descriptors, which may be valid in certain circumstances for a period of time.

In occupational therapy texts 'theory' is often used as an umbrella term to indicate all the *concepts, facts, assumptions* and *hypotheses* on which the practice of occupational therapy is based. A *'theoretical model'* is one which describes some of these ideas and their relevance to practice. (For a discussion of theory in relation to occupational therapy, refer to Miller 1993 and Reed 1998.)

WHERE DOES THEORY COME FROM?

Any profession is informed and shaped over time by a variety of influences both internal and external.

As shown in Figure 2.1, the knowledge and research base of occupational therapy combines with its adopted values, attitudes and ethics and continued input from practical experience to form a stable central core of basic knowledge and practice. This is further enriched by an additional belt of relevant theories drawn from other areas of knowledge (Young & Quinn 1992). This dynamic interaction is continually challenged and modified by the environment of practice.

In this chapter and the next this model will be used to provide a structure for the discussion of the elements which shape theory and practice.

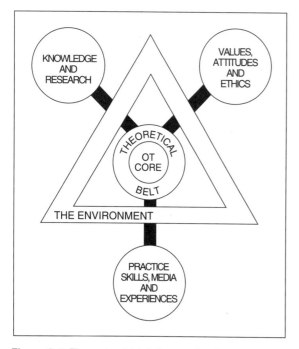

Figure 2.1 Elements which influence the development of theory and practice.

COPING WITH THE TERMINOLOGY USED TO DISCUSS THEORY

The language used to discuss theory can be opaque and intellectually inhibiting, full of 'ists, 'ologies' and 'isms'. Theorists, like all specialists, have developed their own jargon. It is important for the student to make an initial effort to understand the meaning of terms. Use good dictionaries; refer to glossaries.

Just as you do when approaching a foreign language, you need to persevere with translation but also with using the words yourself until you become comfortable with them. To assist you I have included some key definitions in the text and an expanded glossary of theoretical terms at the end of this book (words which are included in the glossary are given in italics).

The language which a professional uses to communicate ideas to others in the same profession is, inevitably, specialized and not readily accessible to outsiders. Having mastered a professional vocabulary the therapist also has to master the art of using it appropriately and selectively, and must be able to explain things 'in plain English' when communicating with clients and others who have no need to be burdened with academic jargon.

EXTERNAL INFLUENCES: THE ENVIRONMENT OF PRACTICE

We tend to concentrate on what happens inside our own profession. Bearing in mind the way in which the environment impedes or enhances our clients' abilities to be competent performers, we should, perhaps, pay more attention to the fact that we are equally dependent on, and influenced by, external conditions. In this chapter I explore some of the significant external influences which have shaped the development of our ideas.

External influences are generated by the environment of practice which includes physical, social, cultural, philosophical, political and economic factors, and developments in what people know, what they do and how they do it.

THE INFLUENCE OF PHILOSOPHY

Opposing views of reality

You may wonder why I begin a discussion of the external influences on the profession with a topic as obscure as philosophy. There are three reasons.

Firstly, it is important to recognize that there are some fundamentally different philosophical perspectives which underpin the various theories concerning human beings and their environment. In particular, there are two opposing *paradigms*, the reductionist paradigm and the holistic paradigm which present very different ways of looking at the world. Many of the misunderstandings which arise when first studying theory spring from a failure to take account of this.

Secondly, when looking at the literature on models and frames of reference, we need to understand where these fit in to the different world views, and how, consequently, the explanation about how individuals function, and what therapists can do to enable occupational performance is altered.

Thirdly, as we will see in Chapter 3, occupational therapy draws on knowledge from both world views. This has left it in an uncomfortable position, straddling 'the great divide'.

During the second half of the 20th century the attempt to reconcile the fundamentally incompatible points of view within its own body of knowledge has swayed the profession first in one direction and then the other, and has occasionally dropped it into the chasm of confusion which lies between.

An understanding of how this confusion originated, and what we may do about it, helps us to criticize and evaluate available models, and decide whether or not they are compatible with occupational therapy.

What is philosophy?

The simple definition of *philosophy* is: 'seeking after wisdom or knowledge, especially that which deals with ultimate reality or with the most general causes and principles of things and ideas and human perceptions and knowledge of them' (Concise Oxford Dictionary).

When a profession's philosophy is described this means something a little different from the above definition. It implies that a profession has a set of beliefs and ideas which it has adopted as a basis for academic development and professional practice. The profession's values, principles and form of practice ought to be in accordance with its philosophy.

There are numerous ways of understanding and exploring the world and our reactions to it. Imagine a beautiful antique pocket watch, the kind in a fine, round gilded case, with an intricate, superbly crafted jewelled mechanism.

From a practical, functional point of view it is simply an object which enables you to measure time with an acceptable degree of accuracy. Alternatively you might consider the watch aesthetically as a thing of beauty. You could try to discover its history, finding out about its maker or the people who have owned it, and what it may have meant to them. You could take it apart into its components of springs and cogs and levers to find out how it is made and how it works. As a physicist you might be able to explore the molecular structure of the metals of which it is composed or investigate the concept of 'time'. Each approach will provide a different understanding of the watch. To know 'all about the watch' you might have to explore them all.

Just as one may understand the watch by looking at it in different ways, so one may understand an aspect of the world, or something about a person, by using different theoretical approaches and perspectives. The theoretical basis of occupational therapy provides these approaches.

DIFFERENT APPROACHES TO KNOWLEDGE

The study of knowledge is called *epistemology*. The view of what knowledge is, how it may be gained, and how language can be used to describe it has changed radically in the course of the last hundred years.

Two significant perspectives governing the search for knowledge are called the *reductionist* (atomist) point of view, and the *holistic* (or organismic) point of view. These have been described as *metamodels* (Reed 1984) since all the other OT models or frames of reference can be viewed as falling into one or other category.

When it comes to getting to grips with difficult philosophical ideas through simplified presentations readers are advised to be cautious. The whole exercise of attempting to put philosophical concepts into 'headlines' or neat pigeonholes and tidy tables (as in Box 2.1) is inevitably liable to oversimplify some very complex thinking.

The following explanations deal with some key ideas and are aimed at providing a general understanding of the issues.

Rationalism and reductionism

At the beginning of the 20th century, when occupational therapy was first evolving, most educated people in Britain and Europe (some philosophers excepted) were confident that the 'big questions' about the nature of humankind, the world, its creatures, and the wider universe had 'answers'. There were fundamental facts and truths, which would sooner or later be discovered. Scientists and researchers of all disciplines had already made so much progress; more was simply a matter of time, analysis and the application of rigorous scientific method. This view is usually referred to as *rationalism* or *logical positivism*.

The scientist usually seeks to understand the nature of objective reality by breaking things down into their component parts. The whole may be understood by studying the components and their functions and structures, and reducing these to the smallest units. Through this analytical and logical process scientific facts and principles may be discovered. This approach is known as *reductionism*.

This process can only be applied to things which have some objective reality or capacity for being examined and measured. Because of this, hard-line reductionists tend to ignore the subjective elements of experience, either as 'unknowable' and therefore not capable of being studied or because they are fundamentally irrelevant. For much of the 20th century research in science and medicine has been based on quantitative, reductionist principles. This is often associated with a *mechanistic* view of human beings; like the pocket watch, the body is a 'machine' which can be broken down into its component parts to find out how it works.

Holism

The *holistic* viewpoint considers things from both objective and subjective perspectives. A thing is an entity which is greater than the sum of its parts; the elements of which it is composed lose meaning when separated from one another. If you dismantle the pocket watch into pieces it remains interesting, but it no longer functions as a watch. The components have not changed, but their meaning is altered.

Abstract and concrete elements interact to form a total *gestalt*. Living organisms interact with each other and their environment, forming complex and dynamic systems the elements of which cannot be understood in isolation from each other.

We live in a world experienced and filtered through our perceptions. Individual experience is valuable. The qualitative aspects of experience are as (or more) important as the quantitative ones. This approach has been influential in education and the social sciences, and in human ecology and anthropology.

Humanism

Humanism originated as a 19th century philosophy which rejected fundamentalist interpretations of the Bible and the notion of an omnipotent deity and saw man as central to human concerns. This is not usually what is meant when the word *humanistic* is used by OT theorists. In OT, humanism is more about the person-centred ethics and values which humanistic psychologists, educators and psychotherapists have introduced during the second half of the 20th century.

Postmodernism

By the end of the 20th century we have learned that almost everything in our universe is far more complex than could ever have been imagined, and much less certain. The optimistic expectation of 'a right answer' has been replaced by the recognition that knowledge depends on the knower, and that there may be several answers, all 'right' (even when they appear to contradict each other). Established facts can be explained in different ways, deconstructed, given a different meaning. This approach may loosely be termed *'postmodern'*.

The study of *meaning*, emotive, descriptive and linguistic, is shared by philosophers and psychologists – one can get quite tangled up in arguments over 'the meaning of meaning'!

Phenomenology

Imagine that I stand on one side of a giant cube with differently coloured sides and you stand on the other. Let us accept that we and the cube exist as real objects in real time. However, we stand in different places and see different things. I will describe seeing a blue square; you will say that you see a red one. We are both correct, but each of us sees only a portion of the cube. The whole is something different, more complicated. If you are colour blind or have been raised in an artificial environment from which the colour red and all concepts connected with it have been excluded, your perceptions will again be different.

What you see changes, depending on where you stand, who you are and your particular view of the world and the way you make sense of it and find meaning in it.

If you study the world in this way you are concerned with *phenomena* – things which can be perceived by the senses. *Phenomenology* is an important 20th century philosophical movement. Like many philosophical movements it has evolved a complex set of ideas concerning consciousness, the nature of our perceptions, and the nature of 'self'. The term 'phenomenological' is also used rather loosely in OT literature to indicate holistic approaches which are concerned with these things.

Where can we look for 'the truth'?

The opposing views of the nature of knowledge have sometimes been expressed as two contrasting statements. The rationalist view is that 'the truth is out there' (that is, unchangeable and waiting to be found).

The postmodern view is that 'the truth is no longer out there'; instead it consists of multiple possibilities within the human mind (Webber 1995; Creek 1997).

Marxism

Marxism is rather different from the schools of thought described so far. Marxist thinking has been very influential in politics and sociology during the 20th century, but it has become entangled with 'left-wing' revolutionary ideals which have obscured much of the original message.

The inclusion of Marxism as an external influence on occupational therapy requires some justification. The link is not Marx's political views concerning capitalism but rather his ideas about the central importance of productive occupation. The following excerpts from a brief explanation of Marx's philosophy make the relevance plain.

Marx viewed human beings as:

Alienated from themselves because their life activity takes an alien, inhuman form. (Marx had in mind monotonous, meaningless industrial tasks.) Truly human and fulfilling activity is an activity of free social self expression ... it is self-determined ... It is the nature of human beings to produce both with others and for others, and to understand themselves in the light of their mutual recognition of one another and their common work ... the ultimate tendency of history is the Promethean drive of the human species to develop its 'essential human powers', its powers of production ... Marx saw the task of the proletarian movement in his time as one of self-definition and growth through organization, discipline and self-criticism based on scientific self-understanding (Honderich 1995).

When these ideas are compared with those expressed by the present generation of OT theorists many similarities of both concepts and language can be detected. It is interesting to speculate how far these theorists are aware of the source of their ideas (Hawes 1996) or whether they have been absorbed without recognizing the originator.

BODY, MIND AND SPIRIT

Another central debate, which has occupied thinkers for several thousand years, concerns whether human beings have a soul or spirit, and how mind and body interact.

Those who believe that humans have both body and mind/spirit and that these are separate entities are known as *dualists*. Those who believe that the mind is inseparable from or a product of body and (usually) that soul or spirit does not exist are called *monists*.

Advances in our understanding of how the brain functions, how language develops and how it may be possible to create artificial intelligence have mainly served to complicate and polarize opinions about the nature and function of the human mind.

Entangled with the dualist/monist argument is the equally ancient debate over whether or not humans have free will and the ability to make choices.

Determinists believe that our actions and choices are inevitable and decided for us by past circumstances or external events (*causality*). This view may be held on scientific grounds; for example, theories that we are programmed to react to the environment in set ways, that our behaviour is genetically determined or that one action inexorably leads to certain others.

This form of determinism is often associated with rationalist or realist approaches and a reductionist, monist perspective.

On the other hand the belief may stem from religious or philosophical ideas about human actions and world history being predetermined by God, fate, the stars or some similar concept. This version of determinism is compatible with dualism. Determinism has interesting consequences for what it means to be responsible for, or ethical about, one's actions.

The opposing view considers humans to have *free will* and to be capable of choosing how to act – for better or worse. This view is usually associated with a more holistic, humanistic, phenomenological perspective which considers thoughts and feelings as well as behaviours. It is also compatible with the idea of spirituality.

KEY SCHOOLS OF THOUGHT ABOUT HUMAN BEHAVIOUR

Humans are far more intricate than a pocket watch and it is therefore inevitable that more than one theory or perspective is required to explain all the complexity and richness of behaviour, thoughts and feelings. The key schools of thought which provide explanations of behaviour are summarized in Box 2.1.

Box 2.1 Key schools of thought concerning human behaviour

Physiological We do what our genetic makeup and electrochemical functions make us capable of doing, in response to internal and external stimuli, in order to maintain homeostasis and satisfy basic survival needs.
Behavioural We perform and react as demanded by the environment. Actions are shaped and modified by the consequences of past behaviour.
Psychoanalytical (classic styles) We act on the basis of infantile drives or experiences and the unconscious memories of past relationships and events.
Cognitive (and cognitive behavioural) We act in accordance with our thoughts, feelings and perceptions.

Developmental We use skills appropriate to our chronological and/or developmental ages, provided that we are given opportunities and a nurturing environment to enable us to do so.
Social We behave as we believe that other people, specific social or cultural groups or society as a whole expect us to behave.
Humanistic We make our own choices about what we do, in accordance with a fundamental respect for ourselves and others.
Ecological We interact with our environment as part of an adaptive, organic, open system. We are shaped by our surroundings and reciprocally shape other parts of the system.

In general the physiological, behavioural and psychoanalytical approaches may be regarded as deterministic and, in various ways, reductive. The rest are holistic.

THE INFLUENCE OF EXTERNAL VALUES, ATTITUDES AND ETHICS

Developments in philosophical thought have, in the past 40 years, filtered through into changes in our values, attitudes and ethics, especially those concerning the role of the individual in society. In particular there has been a radical change – large enough to be regarded as a *paradigm shift*– in views of disability and attitudes towards disabled people.

The biomedical model of disability

The traditional biomedical view of disability was reductionist and somewhat deterministic. It traced the source of the problem to something which had happened to damage the individual (a congenital or developmental problem, an acquired disease or injury) which caused a bodily or mental impairment. An impairment produced some kind of loss or limitation, a disability. This meant the person was handicapped, rendered unable to do things which others could do.

Since there was a causal link between the damage and the consequent disability the action was obvious: treat the patient, 'cure' the condition, remove or reduce the impairment and disability and handicap would consequently be reduced or removed.

Whilst in some cases this linear 'cause and effect' model does indeed hold good it has numerous flaws.

This model was widely accepted during the 1960s and 1970s. The classic approach of physical rehabilitation is based on it. However, the model has a number of disadvantages. For one thing disability is a far more complex phenomenon than this model suggests.

In addition, built into the model are a number of negative attitudes concerning the nature of disability, the degree to which one can do

> **Q** Try to analyse the disadvantages and advantages of the biomedical model from the point of view of patients and practitioners.

> **Q** Analyse the implications of the social model of disability for the individual, society and health care practitioners.

anything about it and the balance of power between the disabled person, health care professionals and society as a whole. The model fits best in acute medical settings (for critical review of this model see Reed & Sanderson 1992).

It is scarcely surprising that, for a whole raft of both practical, philosophical and political reasons, this model was challenged by disabled people themselves and by health care professionals who were dissatisfied with its limitations.

Social models of disability

The major change in the view of disability came when it was proposed that it is 'society' (factors such as culture, attitudes, physical environment, access to resources) which makes a person handicapped, not the health condition or difficulty by which he or she is affected. This was plainly in direct conflict with the former view. An initial compromise was an attempt to combine this new concept with the medical model: this resulted in the *biopsychosocial model*. In this model disability is not an inevitable consequence of something which has happened to an individual, but a result of a combination of adverse factors in the individual's life, including medical, physical, psychological and social factors. Reed and Sanderson (1992) draw attention to the difficulties and inconsistencies associated with this model.

Finally the social model became focused on the way in which the physical, social, cultural, political and economic environment affected the individual and increased or decreased disability. This is plainly a much more holistic view and one, incidentally, which had been accepted by occupational therapists long before it found favour with everyone else.

Offshoots of this radical change in thinking have been the client-centred rehabilitation model, the community-based rehabilitation model and the independent living movement (see McColl et al 1997).

The social model has profoundly influenced health care.

Classification of disability

For many years the most widely used classification has been the the International Classification of Impairments, Disabilities and Handicaps (ICIDH) which was first published in 1980, based on the medical model of disability. At the time of writing (2000) this is being replaced by a new version – the International Classification of Functioning and Disability (WHO; ICIDH-Beta 2 1999), based on the biopsychosocial model (see Glossary).

This aims to provide a 'unified and standard language and framework for the description of human functioning and disability as an important component of health', and to provide 'a systematic coding scheme for health information systems'. It is intended for use as a statistical, research and social policy tool and, significantly for occupational therapists, as a 'clinical tool in needs assessment, matching treatment with specific conditions, vocational assessment, rehabilitation and outcome evaluation'.

The new version shows the influence of the social models of disability which have just been described. It places more emphasis on the perceptions of the individual and the impact of contextual factors. It is significant that the new classification also appears to have been informed by many ideas which appear in occupational performance models; these certainly predate the revision.

This taxonomy introduces new terms including *activities, participation and environmental factors*. A summary of the most important definitions is given (see Expanded definitions) but readers should refer to current WHO documents as work on refining these concepts is continuing. Having an internationally agreed taxonomy is of

great importance and therapists should use it when they can.

The National Center for Medical Rehabilitation and Research (NCMRR 1993) classification

An alternative taxonomy is that produced by the NCMRR in the USA. This uses the terms:

- Societal limitation
- Disability
- Functional limitation
- Impairment
- Pathophysiology

(Christiansen & Baum 1997).

Attitudinal change

We absorb attitudes and values from our social and cultural surroundings. Eventually, although slowly, changed attitudes prompt changes in behaviour.

It is therefore to be expected that the introduction of the social model of disability, changes in thinking about individual rights, lobbying by pressure groups and new legislation have combined to change attitudes and behaviours across the whole range of health care professions (although some have reacted faster than others).

Influenced by humanistic values, health care, like other aspects of life, now has overtly ethical dimensions which were previously ignored or implicit.

Socio-economic, structural and environmental barriers which increase disability are being removed and disability itself has been redefined. Cultural diversity is acknowledged and valued. Sexual, religious or racial discrimination is prohibited by law.

People are increasingly aware of their rights and (to a lesser extent) responsibilities. Above all, the passive and compliant 'patient' has been transformed into the demanding and selective 'consumer'.

Influence on occupational therapy

Even within occupational therapy, which has always viewed its practice as holistic and individualized, the changes from 'biomedical model mind set' to 'social model mind set' over the past 30 years are noticeable.

Consideration of this prompts a personal reflection. I trained in the early 1960s. Casting my mind back I am astonished to recognize the degree to which some of the information which was presented to us as 'fact' would now be regarded as discriminatory, biased and 'politically incorrect'.

For example, people with learning disabilities were still classified as 'idiots' or 'feeble-minded' and incarcerated in long-stay institutions. I recall a visit to the back wards of such an institution where profoundly handicapped, deformed and behaviourally disturbed individuals were proudly exhibited to us much as one might show off a pet or a strange, dangerous animal in a zoo.

Textbooks on psychiatry described homosexuality (the practice of which was illegal) as an illness or as deviant behaviour.

Doctors were to be regarded with subservient respect. The relationship between patient and therapist was mostly framed on the medical model in the classic tradition of 'you come to me so that I can tell you what is wrong with you and what to do to get better'. Therapy was prescribed.

This does not mean that my teachers were consciously discriminatory; they simply taught us the accepted ideas of the day. The fact that 30 years later some of this sounds as out of date as the thinking which inspired the persecution of witches in the 17th century is itself instructive.

(I hasten to add that I was also given an excellent grounding in the principles and practice of occupational therapy, albeit limited by the constraints of what we now called the behavioural, psychodynamic and biomechanical applied frames of reference.)

A limited view

The ideas presented in this chapter are influential, and there are no doubt others which have had some impact on OT. It is important to recognize, however, that almost all these ideas are derived from western occidental thinkers, European or American. Eastern philosophies or those from other countries (for example Africa, South America) have not been included.

This means that the philosophical basis and value system of occupational therapy are culturally biased. It is important to take account of this when transferring these principles into cultures which do not have the same background.

Other external influences

Developments in health care and technology

Changes in medical and surgical practices continually impact on the work of the therapist. They not only alter what is done, but also where it happens and the length of time available for it to be done. There can be no doubt that such changes will continue to alter the scope of occupational therapy.

As health care has evolved other health care professions have also adapted, extended or changed their roles. Occupational therapists typically work in settings where interdisciplinary or multidisciplinary teamwork is important. Changes in the roles of others inevitably affect the role of the OT and create pressures to move in specific directions which may or may not be compatible with the profession's core principles and practice.

Other developments, such as the information technology revolution, do not have such a direct impact, but will inevitably affect practice.

Socio-economic change

The Canadian occupational performance model (CAOT 1997) states that therapists operate at several levels: with the client, within a service and in the context of society. At each of these levels socio-economic factors have significant impact.

For the clients the socio-economic context of their lives can have a real effect on occupational performance (Sussenberger 1998). The gap between 'haves' and 'have nots' is as persistent as it ever was. In the affluent Western world it has, perhaps, been redefined; the starting point is different. In less fortunate areas of the world poverty, exacerbated by political corruption, civil war and natural disaster, still means having insufficient of the basic resources which sustain life.

In the UK the changing structure of society and the diminished role of the nuclear or extended family have weakened support networks and created new forms of isolation and new care needs.

At the level of service delivery the work of the therapist is directly affected by the available resources and the associated systems and structures.

At the level of society, political and economic conditions impact on the delivery of health and social care.

The influence of these contextual factors is important, and requires consideration. Therapists have been rather slow to realize this: OTs tend on the whole to be apolitical.

The chief fact of 21st century health and social care is that resources are never enough to do everything. The increased expectations of the public, changing demography, advances in medicine and technology all combine to force difficult decisions to be taken about what can be provided and what cannot. This leads to numerous practical, ethical, social and political dilemmas.

The consequence of this is that what is done must be demonstrated to be necessary, effective and an efficient and economical use of the available resources. This has challenged all health care professions to undertake more research and to provide evidence-based services (Bury & Mead 1998).

In the UK the concept of clinical governance has been introduced (COT 1999; Sealey 1999) and the recently formed National Institute of Clinical Excellence is charged with ensuring that what is done is worth doing and that it is done well.

Structures and systems have become important, leading to improved techniques of case management, definition of care pathways, methods of audit and quality assurance and attempts to integrate and streamline service provision.

This has further challenged professions to improve basic professional education and to engage subsequently in reflective practice, and a life-long commitment to active learning to ensure that high standards are maintained.

Occupational change

We are accustomed to look at the differences between our own occupations and those of our grandparents as a matter of nostalgic interest or perhaps as a measure of how much things have 'improved' in the sense of being easier, quicker and more efficient. Indeed the occupational differences between ourselves and our forebears at the turn of the century are striking, especially in the case of women. Mountains of paper have been devoted to that topic.

It is plain that people in the developed countries have become very detached from their distant roots in a past where work by hand in close contact with real environments was the norm. Perhaps events are moving too swiftly for us to be able to adapt our skills and our mental processing as we have in the past.

Humanity may soon be forced to pay for this in terms of occupational alienation, occupational deprivation and occupational imbalance (Wilcock 1999a). This problem is not new: it is worth reminding ourselves that Marx recognized occupational alienation as long ago as the 1920s.

It is doubtful whether, as therapists, we have really appreciated the magnitude of these changes or the accelerated pace of change which now confronts us and the impact this will have on the patterns of occupation of our clients, the meanings they derive from them, and the range of media and skills available to us.

SUMMARY

During the past one hundred years new philosophies have had widespread influence on the way we seek to understand ourselves and the world we live in.

Some of these ideas have caused us to change our attitudes and adopt new systems of values and ethics, especially in the areas of health and social care.

Occupational therapy has inevitably been affected by these changes, which have from time to time challenged its fundamental principles and methods of practice.

The health care consumer has become powerful, obliging a review of the therapeutic relationship and models of practice.

In addition the profession has been influenced by the prevailing socio-economic climate and political priorities in health and social care.

Finally and importantly, our profession focuses on human occupation. Consequently the changes in the things people do, the roles they have, and the environments they use affect our practice and our concepts.

3

DEVELOPMENT OF THEORY: INFLUENCES FROM WITHIN THE PROFESSION

As shown in Figure 2.1 OT has a central core of principles and practice surrounded by a belt of additional knowledge drawn from sources external to the profession.

In Chapter 2 we explored some of the philosophical ideas and ways of looking at people which have influenced the content of both belt and core, and noted other external influences on professional development.

In addition the development of theory is influenced by a dialogue between the realities of practice, the values and attitudes held by the profession, advances in professional knowledge and evidence from research.

HISTORICAL PERSPECTIVE

A profession develops over a period of time. It has a history. Understanding the origins of occupational therapy and tracing the course of its subsequent evolution help us to understand the sequence of conceptual development which occurred in parallel with the development of practice.

Evolution during the 20th century

The founders

There is no precise date to pin down the foundation of OT. Some ideas and practices were current in the 19th century, and some aspects can be traced back (albeit somewhat tenuously) to ideals in ancient Greece.

Occupational therapy as we know it originated in America in the early years of the 20th century. The name was coined by George Barton in 1914. The founders were a disparate and at first unconnected group of people from different professions and backgrounds: social workers, psychiatrists, nurses, architects, doctors and craftspeople.

Occupational therapy was introduced to the UK during the 1930s and into Europe and the rest of the world mostly after the Second World War. (For a summary of the history of OT in America and information about some of the founders refer to Miller & Walker 1993, Schwartz 1998. For information on the development of OT in the UK refer to Turner et al. 1996, Tyldesley 1999.)

The founders shared a view of occupation as fundamentally important to human health and well-being, having the potential to be 'curative' if correctly and selectively used. These ideas were generally far ahead of their time.

The breadth of knowledge brought to the profession by these pioneers has been both its strength and its problem. The heritage of ideas and skills drawn from science, medicine, nursing, design, the arts and the humanities has enabled therapists to take a holistic view of the human condition, but at the same time has laid it open to criticism of being 'all breadth and no depth' or 'insufficiently scientific'.

The attempt to combine knowledge from biomedical and psychological reductive and deterministic perspectives with other, more holistic concepts drawn from social sciences and the arts created a built-in philosophical inconsistency which has troubled the profession ever since.

A developmental sequence

It is possible to trace a developmental sequence in the acquisition of knowledge which helps to explain why we have had some difficulty in organizing our conceptual framework. This sequence appears to be replicated in the USA, Canada, Australia, and the UK, although not necessarily at the same time.

To begin with therapists inevitably depended on external sources for their knowledge and skills; there was a theoretical belt but no real core.

They drew on the contemporary understanding of anatomy, physiology, medicine and psychology and acquired skills selected from the practice of teachers, craftspeople, designers and artists.

By the 1930s the body of knowledge required in order to study OT was well defined. An attempt had been made to state a philosophy (Meyer 1922) but for practical purposes the curriculum was expressed mainly in terms of 'things to know and things to do'. Theory was not generally conceptualized as a unique collection of ideas related to the profession.

As practice developed, therapists, ever adaptive, began to modify both knowledge and skills to provide more effective therapy. At the same time a body of practice unique to occupational therapy developed. Practitioners shared ideas and began to build a professional identity on the basis of their experiences.

The Second World War disrupted professional development, but provided stimulus to advances in medicine and psychiatry. By the 1960s therapists in America were becoming concerned with the need to 'create a core' – to provide a rationale for practice, and to formalize the conceptual foundations and body of knowledge.

At this point, influenced by the strongly reductive philosophy at that time permeating science and research, the profession came under pressure to conform to the 'scientific' biomedical paradigm. During the 1960s and 1970s there was a consequent move away from creative, craft-based activities and holistic concepts of occupation.

With hindsight we can detect a division within the profession. Ordinary practitioners increasingly followed the scientific biomedical paradigm and sought to make practice 'more specific', using a variety of frames of reference. Forward thinking OT educationalists and theorists such as Gail Fiddler or Mary Reilly saw the need to move away from borrowed knowledge and to identify theories and principles originated within and serving to define OT.

By the mid 1980s graduate education of occupational therapists was available, promoting a critical, more academic approach to the theoretical foundations of the profession. At the same time the move towards the adoption of a social model of disability was under way. This made holistic approaches more mainstream and acceptable; however, it highlighted the tension between reductionist and holistic models within the profession.

The search for the core culminated during the 1980s with the publication of the first generation of models of human occupation such as those proposed by Kathlyn Reed and Sharon Sanderson (1980 onward) or Gary Kielhofner (1980 onward) (see Section 4).

Too many words!

Description of theory is relatively recent in occupational therapy. The language has had to evolve along with the concepts, and this has caused problems. Theorists have tended to develop their own *taxonomies*, each somewhat different from those of the others.

British and American authors differ from each other, and this is only in part due to the differences between American English and British English.

In textbooks written between 1980 and the late 1990s words such as *paradigm, model, frame of reference* and *approach* were used interchangeably and with different meanings by various authors. This added considerably to the confusion of therapists and students trying to get to grips with the conceptual foundation of practice for the first time. A similar confusion exists over other key words such as *occupation, task* and *activity*.

There have been some interesting, but largely inconclusive debates in the professional literature over which terms should or should not be used.

This is intellectually stimulating, but not of much help to the student who is trying to compare texts and to make sense of complex ideas.

It must sometimes seem as if the student is in a similar position to Alice in her famous exchange with Humpty Dumpty:

'There's glory for you!' 'I don't know what you mean by "glory"', Alice said. 'I meant, "there's a nice knock-down argument for you!"' 'But "glory" doesn't mean "a nice knock-down argument"' Alice objected. 'When *I* use a word,' Humpty Dumpty said in a rather scornful tone, 'it means just what I choose it to

mean - neither more nor less.' (Lewis Carroll, *Alice Through The Looking Glass*)

A review of the conflicting use of language in the past is interesting to the academic but not, perhaps, very helpful to the student seeking a basic understanding of theory. A comparison of the use of the words 'paradigm', 'model', and 'frame of reference' by a selection of theorists between 1984 and 1994 is included to illustrate the problem (Tables 3.1, 3.2). Students who wish to explore further can refer to other texts.

In recent years the controversy has died down, perhaps in part because it has been realized that the semantic debate tends to lead away from the central issue of finding appropriate models and putting them into practice. Authors all acknowledge that there are no fixed definitions and on the whole they appear to have 'agreed to disagree'. Each author decides on a set of terms for a particular publication and a particular system of organizing their material.

For example, in the ninth edition of Willard and Spackman (Neistadt & Crepeau 1998) the authors describe 'theories that guide practice' from several perspectives (occupational behaviour, rehabilitation, infant and child development, learning). Some of these theories are called 'frames of reference', whilst others are described as models. Contributers to Christiansen and Baum (1997) have mainly settled on the term 'model'. My own terminology and structure are different again.

The student must be aware that words are still being used by different people with different meanings. It is useful to have a definition of the terms used in a specific text (and this is not always provided). Where a clear definition is absent students may need to provide their own.

It is unfortunate that internationally recognized standard definitions of descriptive terms and concepts used in occupational therapy do not exist. This flexible use of terminology is unsatisfactory in terms of the profession's need to articulate theory with clarity. I will therefore use my own taxonomy and definitions and give a personal view of the way in which these relate to the development of theory. If you are interested in comparing other views you will need to do further reading.

Table 3.1 Comparisons of terminology used to describe theory: American sources

Source	Paradigm	Model & examples	Frame of reference & examples
Reed (1984)	Discussed in detail. Not the same as model or theory, both 'may be contained within a paradigm'. Explains phenomena; comprehensive: new ideas; ideas for research.	Describes model building in detail. 'conceptual or theoretical models are subtype … which relate to theory building and explanation…' Reed provides list of models too long to quote.	Gives various definitions. 'involves a mechanism which leads to development and use of a standard, schema or set of facts to judge, control or direct some action or expression.' 'A frame of reference is not a model but does form part of the model building process … it explains the relationship of theory to action.'
Mosey (1986)	(Philosophical assumptions and model) Does not use term *paradigm*.	(see paradigm) 'defines and delineates the broad outlines of the profession'.	'delineates a particular area or aspect (of OT) – links model and practice.' Analytical developmental (Recapitulation of ontogenesis) Acquisitional
Kielhofner (1992)	Paradigm 'Core assumptions; focal viewpoint; values → fundamental nature and purpose of OT'.	Conceptual practice models. 'presents and organizes theoretical concepts used by OTs; expresses theory unique to OT'. Biomechanical Cognitive disabilities Cognitive perceptual Group work Model of human occupation Motor control (e.g. Bobath, PNF) Sensory integration Spatiotemporal adaptation	
Hopkins & Smith (1993)	Paradigm (discussed as one name for 'intervening mechanism between theory and practice').	Synonym for paradigm (as Mosey).	Defined as Mosey 'four hierarchical components: theoretical base; function-dysfunction continuum; behaviours indicative of function/dysfunction; postulates regarding change'. Behavioural Biomechanical Cognitive disability Developmental Neurodevelopmental Sensory integration Model of human occupation Rehabilitation Psychodynamic Spatiotemporal adaptation Occupational adaptation

The belt and core: a sequence of conceptual development

The historical development of OT in the USA can be related to the development of a set of basic theoretical concepts. These are widely described under a variety of labels.

When the confusing language is stripped away it becomes possible to identify six distinct concepts concerning the theoretical foundations

Table 3.2   Comparisons of terminology used to describe theory: British sources

Source	Paradigm	Model & examples	Frame of reference & examples	Approach
Young & Quinn (1992)	Discusses scientific origins of term but does not describe an 'OT paradigm'. Describes a 'hard core' of OT knowledge with a 'protective belt' of optional, useful theories.	Function of model: 'framework for complex data; visualization of phenomena; communication of ideas; predictions about real world; stimulates development of theories'.	Functions: 'It specifies the nature, aims and procedures of the work and the features which distinguish it from other forms of practice; it suggests that some theories are more relevant to practice than others'. Adaptive performance Developmental Sensorimotor Cognitive Role performance Rehabilitation	
Turner (1992)	Describes philosophy and values. 'A paradigm imposes shape upon a science. It derives from profession's shared values, principles and knowledge and determines the scope and boundaries of the profession, guiding practice, research and development.' 'provides a general structure for thought'.	'Conceptual model represents basic theories behind practice, delineating the framework for action … and displays links between theory and practice.' Model of human occupation Developmental Occupational performance	'organized body of knowledge, principles and research findings which forms the conceptual basis of a particular aspect of practice – explains relationship between theory and practice.' Humanistic Mosey's 3 F of R (see Table 3.1) Biomechanical Compensatory (Rehab) Learning	'ways and means of doing, i.e. implementing frames of reference'
Creek (1992)	Proposes OT paradigm 'an agreed body of theory explaining and rationalizing professional unity and practice … incorporates all the profession's concerns, concepts and expertise, and guides values and commitment.'	'Simplified representation of structure and content … that describes or explains complex relationships between concepts.' Activities therapy Communication Developmental Model of human occupation	'The principles behind practice; the organization of knowledge in a particular field to permit description of the relationships between facts and concepts.' Psychodynamic Behavioural Developmental Humanistic Adaptive performance Biodevelopment Developmental Occupational behaviour	

of occupational therapy which occur in somewhat different forms in most texts.

Concept 1 Borrowed knowledge

This is knowledge which has been generated by sources external to the profession, but which is applicable to OT practice. This was the first kind of knowledge to be integrated into the profession's core, and it continues to be added to the conceptual belt. There are two related forms of 'borrowing'.

Borrowed science: Basic sciences such as anatomy, psychology, sociology, anthropology, medicine and health sciences provide explanations of function and dysfunction and human behaviour and give the scientific basis for and justification of practice.

Borrowed skills: (which may carry with them related theories) include teaching, counselling, psychotherapy, some physiotherapy techniques, arts and technical skills.

I use the term *primary frame of reference* (PFR) to identify borrowed knowledge which is used in OT with little or no alteration. The most important primary frames of reference are the *physiological PFR* (describing the functions of the human body), the *psychological PFR* (describing the functions of the human mind) and the *educational PFR* (see Section 2).

Concept 2 The OT version

A synthesis of elements of borrowed knowledge together with ideas which have evolved within the profession and the practical experience of providing OT, usually in a speciality, can form a coherent guide to practice. This may be called a frame of reference, model or approach.

I use the term *applied frame of reference (AFR)* to describe these widely used constructs (see Section 2). Examples include the *biomechanical, neurodevelopmental, cognitive and humanistic AFRs*.

Concept 3 Pure OT

A second generation of models of practice have been developed by occupational therapists, for occupational therapists, from around 1980 onwards. These usually explain human occupation and the dynamics of occupational performance. These have been called models and frames of reference.

I describe these as *OT models* or by the generic title *person-environment-occupational performance models* (PEOP model) (see Section 4). A model ought to bring together a collection of ideas in a way which explains, simplifies and integrates theory with practice. OT models are not always successful in achieving all these aims.

Concept 4 Making it work

Theory is of little use unless it can be put into practice. This means that an applied frame of reference or OT model must bring with it a style of relationship with the client and a set of assessments, techniques, procedures and media.

Following common usage in the UK I refer to the application of a model or frame of reference as *an approach*. A summary of frames of reference and associated approaches described in this book is given in Box 8.1.

Concept 5 Processes of change

An individual is able to change sequentially over time. The processes which stimulate change are normal and natural. Occupational therapists seek to take advantage of such processes to enable their clients to move towards specified goals.

These processes, which are a form of borrowed knowledge since they are widely applicable, have been very influential in OT theory building and in practice and they do not fit neatly into any of the previous categories.

These natural processes are:

- Development: the process of maturation and subsequent use of innate potential.
- Adaptation: change in response to external circumstances which is useful to the individual and promotes well-being and survival.
- Education: the process through which the individual learns and acquires knowledge, skills and values.

These are such important processes that one might legitimately describe each as a separate paradigm, having its own set of frames of reference and approaches.

In addition there is an artificial process used by therapists. This is *rehabilitation*, the means of assisting a patient to recover following illness or injury, and to compensate for residual dysfunction. Arguably, rehabilitation can be regarded as a model, but to me it appears more like an organizing framework for the integration of other processes of change and the use of a variety of approaches. It has a particular set of concepts and principles and it is therefore included with the other processes of change in Section 3.

Concept 6 The grand design

There was an attempt (between approximately 1985 and 1995) to provide an overview of OT, describing its philosophy, principles, assumptions, values and beliefs and the nature of its practice (and, by exclusion, a definition of what it is not). This may be referred to as a paradigm, OT model, professional model or core principle.

I refer to this concept as the OT *paradigm*. Paradigm is a contentious word, so its use requires justification. Thomas Kuhn, in his seminal work on the philosophy of modern science, proposed that a paradigm is a set of governing, unquestioned beliefs which underpin practice and research.

He suggested, controversially, that at intervals a paradigm is challenged by new evidence. If the new ideas are accepted the old paradigm may be demolished, and replaced by a new one. (For example, the paradigm that the world is flat and the centre of the universe was challenged on the basis of astronomical observations and calculations and replaced by the concept that the world is round and circles the sun.) (Honderich 1995 provides a brief summary of the ideas of Kuhn and other philosophers.)

It is debatable whether occupational therapy has a paradigm of this type, but it does have a paradigm in the more general sense of a pattern or template, a set of underlying principles and beliefs which change only slowly over time. I prefer to use paradigm rather than 'professional model' in order to distinguish between a higher and more comprehensive level of theory and the kind of theories which are applied in practice.

Terminology used in this book

I have analysed these underlying concepts to provide a set of terms to distinguish between the different kinds of theory.

Box 3.1 summarizes the concepts and terms used in this book.

Relationships between the concepts

It is tempting to arrange these concepts as a hierarchy, moving from theory towards practice as

Box 3.1	Concepts and terms used in this book	
Concept		**Term**
Concept 1:	Borrowed knowledge	Primary frame of reference
	Borrowed skill	
Concept 2:	The OT version	Applied frame of reference
Concept 3:	Pure OT	OT PEOP model
Concept 4:	Making it work	Approach
Concept 5:	Processes of change	Processes of change
Concept 6:	The grand design	Paradigm (syn. Professional model)

suggested by Kortman (1994). The relationship is not, however, a simple one. Figure 3.1 shows only some of the interactions.

The knowledge derived from external sources finds its way into the OT paradigm and also into applied frames of reference and OT models. These provide practical approaches for service delivery.

Theorists within the profession work within the boundaries of the paradigm to develop applied frames of reference and OT models. Feedback loops from the results of practice inform and subtly alter the paradigm (though without altering fundamental principles) and result in the development of new concepts and approaches.

Provided all the elements can be kept in balance within the framework of critical evaluation and reflection, the result is an organic and dynamic evolution of practice.

OTHER INTERNAL INFLUENCES

Having explored the way in which theoretical concepts have evolved during the 20th century, we must review the other internal influences on professional development. As shown in Figure 2.1 these are: the profession's values, attitudes and ethics; the skills and techniques used in practice; the developing knowledge and research base of the profession.

Values, attitudes and ethics

Humanistic values

We have seen how the attitudes and values of society as a whole have been changed by the

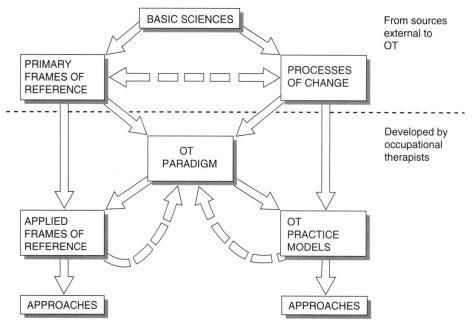

Figure 3.1 Relationships between the concepts.

acceptance of a social model of disability, and by other humanistic ideas.

Occupational therapists have probably always been client-centred, in the sense of being focused on an individual and his needs, but in the past five years they have consciously opted for client-centred models and forms of practice.

The provision of therapy has been transformed into the client-led process of enablement and empowerment, with an associated set of values. (For lists of values see Hagedorn 1995a, Townsend 1997.)

Recent texts discuss these ideas using concepts and language which will not be found in books published only a decade earlier (e.g. Christiansen & Baum 1997 (Chapter 2 and Section 3); Neistadt & Crepeau (Unit 11) 1998; Wilcock 1998a, b; Law 1998).

It may sound heretical to question these ideals but there is a problem. As noted in Chapter 2, occupational therapy has evolved in the context of Western socio-economic values and resources and reflects contemporary attitudes to the individual's expectations of personal wealth and his right to achieve a high level of well-being and opportunities for self-actualization.

We should, perhaps, challenge some of our values and assumptions to test whether they are applicable in cultures and environments which differ from those in which they have evolved. We may sometimes need to use the touchstone of real deprivation to evaluate whether we truly provide services which are essential to human well-being.

Code of ethics

The profession has a strong code of ethics (COT 1997), supported by sanctions against malpractice. Ethics are informed by values and beliefs concerning health, well-being and the role of occupations in maintaining these.

Ethical concerns are never simple. Apart from the usual dilemmas which arise in practice, ethical problems are being generated by issues such as 'rationing' of services, restricted resources, charges for services and the need to set priorities. All of these things can impose limitations on clients' choices and the freedom of the therapist to provide an 'ideal' service (Barnitt 1998).

Empirical factors: input from skills and experience

What we do is informed by our professional knowledge, but what we know is also informed and changed by what we do.

In a practice-based profession skills, media and techniques need to evolve just as much as theory. There remains an important function for discussion: description and communication of the art of practice; and for personal reflection on what is done.

We have to be vigilant to ensure that practice does not become out of step with theory, and that theory takes account of what is actually being done.

Academic development and professional education

Occupational therapists in many countries are now educated at graduate level, and there are opportunities for masters' degrees and doctorates. The quantity and quality of academic literature and research have therefore increased.

Therapists who have moved into professional education have become expert in curriculum development, academic research and educational models and techniques. This has promoted constructive criticism of the OT curriculum, and dialogue with educators from other disciplines. Practitioners who supervise students have also become more aware of educational issues and the necessity of adopting a well-founded rationale for practice.

Continuing research and development

Professional practice continues to be informed by developments in knowledge and the findings of research in other fields. In addition occupational therapists undertake research into both practical and theoretical aspects of their work, testing hypotheses, validating practice and measuring outcomes.

There is no argument over whether research should be done: there is, however, a difference of opinion over the most appropriate research methods. This relates back to the debate over whether it is legitimate to use reductive approaches (and, consequently a quantitative, traditional scientific approach to research) or whether to use qualitative research methods which are more compatible with the holistic nature of practice.

Probably, we need both; just as selecting a therapeutic approach depends on the problem and context, so selection of research techniques depends on the nature of the question and the practical constraints in each situation.

OCCUPATIONAL THERAPY IN THE 21ST CENTURY: WHERE ARE WE NOW?

During the late 1990s, after a great deal of intellectual effort and debate a whole generation of similar occupational performance models emerged, indicating that the profession had reached a consensus view of the fundamental principles of the profession.

These models are all holistic, client-centred and based on social and humanistic views of health and disability. They are rooted in a well-defined set of concepts and assumptions concerning human occupation. These ideas are described in detail in Section 4.

It is unclear whether this general agreement marks the end, for the time being, of the 'search for the core' or merely a point along the way. There are some indications that therapists now want to descend for a while from the heights of abstract conceptualization and return to the more practical aspects of practice.

Maintaining the integrity of the core: a continuing challenge

Knowledge evolves, sometimes slowly and occasionally in leaps and bounds. It is seldom presented gift-wrapped in a neat package. The knowledge which underpins OT has been gained over almost a century of professional development. This slow accretion enriches but it does not always promote coherence.

Occupational therapists are adaptive and acquisitive and open to new ideas. They are not, however, as critical as they might be about the relevance of the knowledge and skills which they draw into professional practice. One cannot manage the core of professional knowledge in the same way as the traditional OT store-cupboard, crammed with 'come-in-handies' which may or may not be of use, and subject to occasional ruthless and indiscriminate spring-cleaning when space runs out.

When the core knowledge of a profession is permitted to absorb external influences indiscriminately there is a risk that it may fragment or mutate into something very different from what it was at the start. If the synchronicity between internal and external influences is lost there may be unwanted side-effects. External sources may become overly influential in shaping practice and may move the profession away from its roots. It may be difficult to decide what is 'belt' and what is 'core'.

Alternatively the profession may become inward looking, busily creating itself in its own image, without regard for the environment of practice or the needs and wishes of service users.

The need for coherence

Practical considerations

You will probably have realized by now that combining techniques from compatible frames of reference is likely to be more effective than attempting to draw eclectically from opposing perspectives.

For example, in its classic form behaviourism is reductionist and deterministic, whereas humanism is based on a holistic view of the person which promotes choice and self-actualization. It would not be effective to use a strict behavioural modification programme, whilst at the same time offering the patient a client-centred programme promoting choice. (Conflicts of this kind are not unknown when different members of a treatment team work on the basis of incompatible models of practice without adequate discussion.)

This is not to say that a skilful and experienced practitioner may not break the rules and succeed in combining incompatible techniques, but this should only be done with full understanding and extreme caution.

Philosophical coherence

There is a more fundamental issue in the selection of an approach. If OT has largely rejected reductionism and determinism, is it legitimate for occupational therapists to use these frames of reference? This problem has not been totally resolved.

Physiological, behaviourist and classic psychoanalytical theories tend to be reductionist and determinist; of these, only the physiological frame of reference is much favoured by occupational therapists in Britain, principally when working in the field of physical rehabilitation. Classic behaviourism and Freudian or neo-Freudian analytical theories are not seen as compatible with contemporary humanistic values and client-centred forms of practice, although they remain as alternatives in specialist areas. The other approaches are all holistic (in various degrees) and are widely used.

Since much of our foundation knowledge is derived from biological, behavioural and medical sciences, we cannot totally reject the reductionist view. But occupational therapists also understand people from sociological and ecological perspectives; they are prepared to explore the intangible, symbolic and irrational aspects of human thought and behaviour.

One way of resolving this paradox may be to adopt the postmodern perspective on knowledge as multifaceted and continually open to deconstruction, leading to new interpretation and description.

Another strategy may be to use the different paradigms at different stages in the intervention process or in relation to different levels of occupation (Hagedorn 2000).

Taking a wider view

The European experience

It is important to note that the development of OT theory in Europe has not followed the American path; or if it has, it is doing so more slowly and by a different route.

There are a number of historical and philosophical reasons for this difference. The Second World War profoundly affected philosophical thinking in Germany, France and other parts of western and northern Europe. Most of the intellectuals who followed theological, phenomenological or humanist schools of thought were persecuted. Some were killed. Those who could left to continue work in America or other countries.

Following this period, health care in several parts of western Europe has been dominated by the medico-scientific reductionist models. OT has used these models and has also been influenced by the work of German and French philosophers and psychologists.

This has meant that many of the concepts which underpin the thinking of American OT theorists were not (and in some cases still are not) generally understood or current in parts of Europe.

Apart from this imposed limitation on ideas, development of other views has been impeded by the inaccessibility of English language texts on OT theory, a few of which are only now being translated. No conceptual models have yet been proposed by European therapists. (Therapists in other non-English speaking countries have similar problems.)

For several years European therapists have been concerned to develop the profession and to overcome intellectual isolation. The Committee of Occupational Therapists in the European Community (COTEC) and the European Network of Occupational Therapists in Higher Education (ENOTHE) are engaged in dialogue and research. They are actively networking within Europe and with other countries. This means that they are now starting to catch up along the development pathway outlined above.

The current state of awareness of theory is indicated by a recent survey of 16 OT schools in 10 European countries. This was conducted by staff at the Portuguese School of Occupational Therapy (Van Bruggen 2000).

This showed that most schools teach the familiar applied frames of reference (much as listed in Section 2 of this book, and no doubt derived from the American and British literature). The most widely taught OT models are the Candian Occupational Performance Model (12) and the Model of Human Occupation (14).

Unfortunately, however, reliance on literature from external sources may have some disadvantages. For one thing the concepts are culturally biased and may not translate well into different contexts. Secondly there is a danger that European therapists (including those in Britain) may be content to let others do the thinking, valuing imported ideas above home-grown ones. This may well deprive the rest of the OT world of some valuable perspectives drawn of different intellectual and cultural traditions.

OT across the world

Occupational therapy is now practised world wide. The coordinating body is the World Federation of Occupational Therapists (WFOT).

Interest in theory is increasing, but has inevitably been dominated by the American academics, whose work has been pioneering and seminal. It is to be hoped that the next generation of therapists will have the confidence to criticize OT models and frames of reference and to produce some of their own, reflecting the cultural diversity and occupational differences in their own countries. A wider world view will enrich practice and promote critical evaluation of fundamental principles.

Occupational science

Complementary to but distinct from the development of OT theory is the evolution of a new area of enquiry, occupational science. This was formalized as an accepted field of study in 1989 when the University of Southern California instituted a doctorate course (USC 1989).

The Journal of Occupational Science Australia (1994) states that occupational science is the rigorous study of:

- The human need to be occupied
- The purpose of occupation in survival and health
- The effects of occupation and occupational deprivation
- Why humans strive for occupational competence and mastery
- What prevents or enhances occupational performance
- How social, cultural and political structures affect occupation
- How occupation provides biological and sociocultural needs
- How occupation is necessary in the development of human capacities.

It is a social science which covers the form, function, meaning and socio-historical context of occupation and explores the occupational nature of human beings. It is strongly phenomenological and anti-reductionist: individuals are viewed as engaging in purposeful, meaningful interaction with their environments, within the stream of past, present and future time. People cannot be decontextualized.

Systems theory has been influential in framing some of the concepts concerning human occupation and, whilst this has introduced some important ideas, it has also, unfortunately, brought with it a somewhat impenetrable vocabulary.

Although the prime movers in the development of occupational science were occupational therapists, the field is interdisciplinary. Those involved include occupational therapists, but also anthropologists, philosophers, psychologists, sociologists, educationalists and human ecologists.

The degree to which occupational science will influence or inform OT is at present unclear. It provides a forum for discussion and research which will certainly enrich our understanding of occupations. It may provide new therapeutic techniques, e.g. occupational story telling (Clark et al 1996).

The importance of experiencing performance as an integrated, spontaneous, meaningful process, rather than a series of detached events, is already challenging more reductive approaches to the therapeutic use of occupation.

Occupational science has stimulated discussion about occupation and particularly the meaning and purpose of human life as expressed through engagement in and reactions to personal occupations (e.g. Nelson 1988, 1996; Trombley 1995a; Wilcock 1993, 1998a, 1998b).

LOOKING TO THE FUTURE

We have explored some of the influences on the development of theory in OT, and it is clear that changes in the environment of practice have a significant effect on both theory and practice. At the start of a new century it seems appropriate to consider whether that environment will be supportive or hostile to the continued evolution of OT.

During the 1990s prominent therapists (Yerxa 1994, Polatajko 1994, Nelson 1997) made statements about the ways in which OT may develop in the 21st century. Although acknowledging that the profession faces decisions and dilemmas, these authors have a positive view of the potential of OT.

However, these statements appear to be based on the premise that life in the 21st century will be a progression from life in the 20th. Things will change, of course, but not out of all recognition. This may not be the case.

As discussed in Chapter 2, we have already seen huge changes in the way we live our lives. Concepts of nationality and national boundaries are altering rapidly. We can travel to most places in a matter of hours, pin-point our location to within a few yards, communicate with anyone, anywhere in seconds. The amount of information already available to us on the World Wide Web is already vastly beyond the capacity of any individual to assimilate and this will increase exponentially.

Bearing in mind the OT view of the importance of environmental demand in shaping our lives and occupations, these developments must bring real changes in our perceptions of ourselves, our world, our relationships to others and the nature of our actions.

The advent of the millennium caused a flurry of media speculation and prediction concerning the possible changes in the new century. Many of these ideas are gloomy and disturbing and some are simply bizarre. These apparent fantasies are not always fringe speculations but the ideas of respected scientists who have proposed them as serious possibilities.

In the foreseeable future, if the genetic revolution lives up to expectations, we may be able to banish many illnesses and grow our own spare parts. We could defeat old age and live for hundreds of years. I find it a matter of concern that few pundits pause to question how we will adapt to an extended life-span and how we will occupy ourselves throughout the promised centuries of healthy living.

At the more extreme end of the predictions industry futurologists have made even stranger suggestions. By the end of this century we may clone ourselves or have 'designer babies' which never need a womb. At least, we may if we are wealthy. Given that genetic technology is unlikely to be universally available, the human race could divide into two species: a genetically perfect minority, healthy and virtually immortal, and the imperfect, unhealthy masses who breed and die in the usual way.

Perhaps we will mutate into beings which are part human, part machine and live our lives in a virtual cyber world. Or maybe super-intelligent machines will take over and relegate us to the status of pets in a zoo (that is, if global warming, a volcanic super-catastrophe or a rogue meteor doesn't get us first!). Escape to a terraformed biosphere on the moon or Mars begins to sound like a good idea.

If even a few of the less apocalyptic prophesies come true it is hard to envisage human life under these conditions. Occupational therapy, as a child of the 20th century, would hardly seem relevant.

If, however, we take a more optimistic stance, where will OT be in 30 or 40 years time? Maybe, just maybe, common sense will prevail and humans will resist the temptation to do things just because they can be done. Perhaps we will find the wisdom to take the best and leave the rest. Then life may go on much as before, but healthier and happier, with people engaged in a balance of meaningful work, leisure and self-care in real environments which they enjoy and strive to protect.

Then occupational therapy will live up to its promise, offering an essential service to enable performance and enrich and enhance people's lives. Who knows? It is certainly going to be a challenging century.

4

CORE PROCESSES USED IN OCCUPATIONAL THERAPY

The wide scope of the work undertaken by occupational therapists has already been described. If an uninformed observer were to see the work of individual practitioners from different specialities there might seem to be, at a superficial level, little in common between them.

The therapist who assesses the home for the provision of an adapted ground floor extension, the one who takes a session of psychodrama and the one who rehabilitates a patient's hand function following a severe crush injury may appear at first glance to be doing very different things.

Is there a common core of practice, a shared understanding of key competencies and processes? If so, can this be described? 'What do we do that is different?' is a central question for any profession.

If the question is not answered it becomes difficult to define the requisite body of knowledge or to specify the standard of competency which students must acquire in order to practise. It is also difficult to define and defend service provision, set and maintain standards, ensure quality or ensure that occupational therapists' skills are used to best effect, which is of increasing importance when resources are stretched and therapists are in short supply.

For these reasons there has been considerable interest, both from the profession and its managers, in identifying and describing core skills and 'skill mix'. This process is not without its dangers. If carried to extremes it may become reductive. The attempt to define the knowledge, skills and values which underpin the profession might lead us to adopt standardized practices and formulae which actually inhibit thinking and dynamic professional development. Therapy might then be considered as a mechanistic process, more at a technical level than that of a graduate professional practitioner.

Our core competencies and processes must somehow encompass the nebulous aspects of professional judgement and reasoning, problem solving and research as well as the 'hands on' forms of therapeutic knowledge and skill.

The terms *core skill* and *competency* occur in the literature and are often used interchangeably. In this text I use the terms to indicate different levels of knowing and doing.

Core   simply indicates that the skill or competency is one of the essential elements of professional practice, the use of which remains relatively constant, although adapted by the selection of therapeutic models or frames of reference.

A skill   is a practised action which may be employed in various situations in different combinations; for example, observing performance, recording information, measuring range of movement, establishing the therapeutic relationship with a client are all skills.

A competency   is a set of skills which are used in a specific context and setting, e.g. using a specific assessment of activities of daily living, running an anger management group, providing a therapeutic programme for a patient who has had a stroke.

A process   is a collection of skills and competencies related to a definable area of OT practice.

Q Before going any further, write down your own list of OT core competencies, the things which are essential for effective practice. Then try to divide your list into things which *only* OTs do, or do in some very specialized way and those which other health care professions may use. If you can, compare your list with someone else's and discuss the similarities and differences.

This exercise will probably demonstrate that it is far from easy to untangle the things which are *only* done by occupational therapists from those which many other professions may do. It is also hard to separate the essential elements from those which may be peripheral or only used in a speciality. It has to be remembered that all such analysis is artificial; in practice therapy is delivered as a total package. Most attempts at defining core skills are made, consciously or unwittingly, from the perspective of the writer's speciality and preferred model of practice which leads us to emphasize particular aspects and to ignore others.

INTERVENTION

The generic and core processes, competencies and skills of occupational therapy, together with core knowledge concerning people, their occupations and their environment, provide the building blocks from which the therapist constructs individualized service provision to assist each client.

Each time a new individual is referred to the therapist the processes must be recombined or synthesized into a fresh arrangement within the overall structure of the OT process, and modified by an applicable theoretical structure.

Therapy simply means treatment; however, therapists these days very rarely 'treat a patient' in the sense of doing something to her with the intention of removing or reducing the impact of an impairment.

In OT action must be taken by the patient or client although it may be initiated or facilitated by the therapist, and the approach is usually focused on the enhancement or restoration of occupational function and competence. The therapist and client work as a team to identify what is needed and then find a means of achieving the stated goals. Ideally the client will be facilitated to take most of the required action. However, there is often the need for some action by the therapist on behalf of the client, such as writing letters, making contact with other agencies which may assist the client, obtaining equipment, planning adaptations, communicating with relatives or making home visits. Studies have estimated that between 30% and 50% of a therapist's time may be spent in actions which are not 'hands on/face to face' therapy. In the case of the community-based therapist these aspects are likely to form the major part of the therapist's work.

The term *intervention* is therefore used to indicate this broadly based form of service provision.

The way in which intervention is shaped and influenced by theoretical structures and approaches is described in the following chapters. First the OT process requires examination.

THE OT PROCESS: A FRAMEWORK FOR INTERVENTION

The OT process is the name given to the sequence of actions which a therapist undertakes in order to provide services to a patient or client. It is not a theory, nor is it therapy; it is a systematic method of organizing practice.

There have been several representations of this process in OT textbooks, each differing a little from the others in accordance with the author's personal concept of the sequence.

In general there is close agreement on the basic format. This involves gathering information concerning the client, her situation and problems, evaluating this information and defining the aims of intervention in close cooperation with the client; setting consequent priorities for action, deciding on how to achieve these, implementing action and evaluating the outcome.

This process is clearly not unique to occupational therapy. It is a form of problem analysis and solution (see page 51) which is used by all health care professionals. For example, the nursing process (Yura & Walsh 1988) consists of four stages: assessing, planning, implementing and evaluating.

As shown in Figure 4.1 a referral is received by the therapist. This starts the intervention sequence. The therapist will then enter the cycle of information gathering and problem analysis, decision making, implementation of action and review of outcome which is repeated until intervention is judged to be completed.

So, if this is a generic process which is used by other professions, what makes it into occupational therapy and not nursing or psychology? The answer is at once very apparent and very complex; it is an occupational therapist who is using the process.

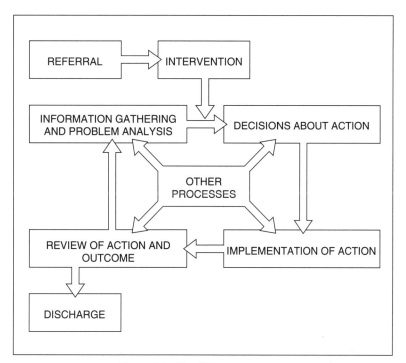

Figure 4.1 The OT process.

The occupational therapist employs the unique combination of personal experience, knowledge, skills and values which form the practice of OT. Because of his training he is able to use the OT process, as directed by his clinical reasoning, to coordinate and combine other processes. The way in which this happens and the manner in which the reasoning process is informed and directed by models of practice are explained in Chapter 5.

GENERIC SKILLS AND COMPETENCIES

It is clear that some of the skills and competencies used by occupational therapists are also used by others. These may be regarded as *generic*, that is, of general application.

Of course each profession may interpret and use these competencies in a slightly different way and in different contexts, but fundamentally what is done is more or less the same. These key generic skills and competencies may be loosely grouped under the headings of management, care of patient/client, and research (see Box 4.1)

Management

Occupational therapists have to manage services, a case load, resources, other people and, importantly, themselves. Management skills are dealt with in many textbooks (Mullins 1993; for an OT perspective, Johnson 1996; Gore 1997).

Box 4.1 Key generic skills and competencies
MANAGEMENT Service management and organization Problem-solving skills Record keeping Communication skills CARE OF PATIENT/CLIENT Observation skills Provision of basic care Handling skills RESEARCH Use information technology Evaluate and develop service provision Communicate results to others

---

A key managerial skill for therapists is the ability to evaluate the outcomes of intervention in order to be able to justify that what is done is efficient, effective, and a good use of resources.

The therapist needs to set standards, monitor quality and audit performance. The findings need to be communicated within the profession and to others. The therapist must be critical of his or her performance, seeking regular supervision and evaluating and updating personal knowledge.

OT managers have become concerned to find means of measuring outcomes: this is more difficult than at first appears, and there is still much debate about how it can best be done.

Care of patient/client

Anyone who works closely with people who may be vulnerable or who have special needs requires a repertoire of skills which are aimed at identifying and meeting these needs appropriately.

The therapist has to use observation skills to take account of the physical appearance of the person. This might include facial expression, posture or dress. She may need to observe external changes of medical significance such as alteration in skin colour, sweating or the condition of a scar. Observation of patterns or frequency of communication and non-verbal signals are important.

People may need personal care such as assistance with walking, eating or use of the lavatory. The therapist must maintain comfort and correct positioning and ensure a safe environment. She must pay attention to safe handling and lifting. Personal rights and dignity must be maintained.

Research

As a graduate the therapist will have an understanding of basic research methodology. As a professional person, she must have a commitment to continual improvement and development of her own practice (life-long learning), and to enhancing and extending the overall knowledge base of the profession. Setting standards and evaluating effectiveness and outcomes are no longer the preserve of a few specialist researchers, but essential skills for all practitioners.

CORE PROCESSES OF OT

Core processes of occupational therapy are described and discussed in detail in my other texts (Hagedorn 1995a, 2000), and the description which follows is therefore only a summary.

Over the decade between 1985 and 1995 some consensus over the core skills or processes of practice became apparent, as shown in Table 4.1. My view is that there are four core processes which combine to form the unique practice of OT. These are:

- Therapeutic use of self
- Assessment of individual potential and skill
- Analysis and adaptation of occupations
- Analysis and adaptation of environments.

Therapeutic use of self

In nursing, social work or the remedial professions, the dyadic therapeutic relationship between the professional and the patient/client is of great importance. The basic skills of listening, observing non-verbal cues and adapting responses are required by all health care practitioners.

Whilst occupational therapists frequently engage in ordinary dyadic interactions, the process of occupational therapy is unique in that the relationship may be considered not as a dyad (therapist/patient) but as a *triad* (therapist/patient/occupation). The occupation/activity is the medium whereby the interaction is enabled or explored.

Whether working with an individual or with a group, the therapist's awareness of personal attributes and skills in interpersonal relationships and the sensitive and empathetic use of such attributes or skills in the context of an activity or task in order to develop a therapeutic relationship with the participant(s), and to achieve a therapeutic goal, is at the centre of the practice of occupational therapy.

The use of this process could include the following skills.

- Select and enhance features of an activity to promote specific interactions.
- Decide on degree of direction/non-direction/leadership style.
- Use knowledge of group process appropriately.
- Allow or restrict personal spontaneity.
- Control use of humour.
- Set limits for self.
- Be aware of own emotions and reactions: consciously use these for positive therapeutic purposes or avoid negative effects on therapy.

Table 4.1 Comparison of lists of core skills

Mosey (1986) (legitimate tools)	Reed (1992) (service provisions)	Hopkins & Smith (1993) (tools of practice)	COT (1994) (skills)
Use of the non-human environment	Use of normal or adapted environments	Environmental adaptation	Assess and manipulate environments
Conscious use of self		Therapeutic use of self	
The teaching-learning process	Teaching		
Use of purposeful activities	Use of normal activities	Use of activity and activity analysis	Therapeutic use of purposeful activity
Use of activity groups	Use of activity groups	Group process	
Activity analysis and synthesis	Use of adapted activities and task analysis	(Activity analysis)	Analysis and application of activities
Assessment and evaluation	Assessment and evaluation Use of adaptive equipment	Assessment and evaluation Assisted and adaptive equipment: use of technology Service management Research	

- Understand own attitudes and prejudices and possible effects on relationships; avoid being judgemental.
- Define and adhere to own meaning of 'professional behaviour' and 'ethics'.
- Monitor self and be aware of own needs.
- Be aware of dangers of manipulating or dominating others.
- Give patient appropriate reactions, e.g. praise, encouragement, consolation.
- Use confidence in self to give patient confidence and trust in treatment.
- Use personal initiative, imagination, creativity.

Assessment of individual abilities and needs

Areas of assessment

Occupational therapists need to understand what an individual *can* do, and evaluate the potential to do more. This is set against the assessment of what difficulties the individual currently experiences in occupational performance in the areas of work, leisure or self-care.

This is further related to the past patterns of participation, and the expectation of future patterns of engagement. To conduct a comprehensive assessment of all these areas is complex and time-consuming. This may not always be necessary; very specific problems require a narrower field of investigation; however, the trend is towards a holistic assessment of abilities and needs.

The areas of assessment in Box 4.2 are well-documented.

In addition, specific frames of reference carry with them assessments of defined areas of performance such as:

- Physical mobility
- Hand function
- Cognitive and perceptual skills
- Social skills
- Intrapersonal (cognitive/affective) skills.

When undertaking an OT assessment it is usual to observe a client performing specified tasks or activities in home, workplace or community environments (or in a well-simulated approximation to the real thing).

Assessment skills

It is acknowledged that the basic skills of assessment (e.g. select what is to be assessed; select or design correct assessment methods; be objective; show good observation skills; produce consistent, accurate and where possible replicable results; communicate results clearly to others; be sensitive to the patient as an individual not an object) are used by other professions but, in the context of OT, a crucial primary core skill is the ability to conduct assessments and to analyse the results in order to plan therapy or intervention in an area of occupational performance or dysfunction. Assessments may be conducted within an applied frame of reference or model or as a means of selecting one.

Assessment should be recognized as a means to an end – identification of the problem; definition of a starting point for treatment/intervention; measurement of progress; evaluation of

Box 4.2 Type of assessment	Occupational area
Functional assessment:	personal activities of daily living, domestic or instrumental activities of daily living (PADL; DADL; IADL)
Work assessment:	work skills; work readiness
Leisure assessment:	participation in social and leisure activities
Participation assessment:	review of overall patterns of past or current activities and lifestyle
Investigation of occupational meaning:	exploration of personal meanings and values connected with roles and occupations, and implications for future goals

outcome – not as an end in itself. There is little value in defining a problem if it is not then possible to offer to do something about it.

Assessment may be formal or informal, be used once or sequentially, and can utilize a wide variety of techniques. Assessment involves:

- Information gathering
- Observation
- Measurement
- Recording
- Evaluation against a norm or outcome.

Assessment methodology

There is extensive literature about the structure and methods of assessment. Assessments need to be valid and reliable.

Validity concerns whether the assessment actually deals with matters which are appropriate to the situation and measures the right things.

Face validity means that it looks as if the assessment does these things, but it has not been proved to do so. Scientific validity has to be tested and proved by formal research involving control groups, using researched and accepted norms of performance, and tested for statistical validity.

Reliability means that you can be sure that, provided the assessment is used correctly each time the test is used (test-retest reliability) and whoever uses it (inter-rater reliability), the results can be depended upon. Gaining evidence of reliability in scientific terms is another difficult and time-consuming process involving much research.

Formats for assessment

Assessments may be:

Standardized – usually conducted following a format which has been piloted on a reasonably large sample of subjects and adjusted for inter-rater reliability. There is an explicit standard against which the results of the assessment can be judged. There are numerous standardized and validated tests on the market, particularly in the areas of cognition, intelligence, perception, personality and performance skills. Some of these would be of use to occupational therapists but can only be purchased following special training.

Informal – ad hoc, unstandardized tests; assessments based on subjective observation in normal environments. Many assessments are constructed by occupational therapists and whilst these employ questionnaires, checklists, grading systems and structured performance tests few are standardized and very few properly validated, not least because this requires detailed research, large samples of patients and control groups, and because it is an extremely complex and time-consuming procedure which is beyond the scope of most busy practitioners.

Single or sequential – an assessment may be a 'one off' exercise or a sequential process where the same performance is reassessed at intervals. In either case there may be a standardized measure or the individual's previous performance or 'normal' performance where this is observable can be used as the base line.

Objective or subjective – it is impossible (outside of laboratory conditions, and perhaps even then) to be totally objective. Some performances can be assessed with reasonable consistency against known criteria, but many cannot. The criteria do not exist; the effects of environment, the therapist/patient relationship, the mood and motivation of the patient, the skills, expectations, attitudes and intentions of the observer and the well-documented effects of the process of being observed on the performance of the subject, all have the potential to alter or at worst invalidate assessment results. In the context of OT, it may have to be accepted that intuitive methods of assessment, based on experience and professional judgement, can be valid.

The patient's understanding of his problem is often revealing, and some assessments are designed to elicit this subjective view.

Assessment procedures

All assessment procedures require a basis of theoretical knowledge and practical experience and expertise. Basic methods may be used in a variety of ways, formal and informal. The subject may be asked to perform an action or complete a task or to complete a self-rating form. Alternatively, the therapist investigates or measures, whilst the subject is relatively passive.

Procedures for obtaining information

- *Interviews*: informal and unstructured or formal and structured.
- *Questionnaires*: self-rating or administered.
- *Performance tests*: physical; cognitive; interactive. The subject completes a task or demonstrates skill or knowledge.
- *Measurement techniques*: frequently of physical function.
- *Observation and sampling techniques*: to obtain a profile of the subject.

Procedures for collating and evaluating information

- *Rating scales*: giving a grading or numerical score.
- *Checklists*: as a structured aid to observation.
- *Record forms*: a structured aid to observation and sequential comparison.
- *Charts, grids or graphs*: a visual aid to recording and evaluating results.
- *Statistical formulae*: to evaluate significance of data.
- *Profiling*: provides a comprehensive 'picture' of the subject.

Analysis and adaptation of occupations

The analysis of occupations and their prescription as therapy are the unique skills of the occupational therapist. The analysis and prescription of occupations have two purposes.

- To deal with problems experienced by the patient in all aspects of his or her everyday life or with social roles (e.g. parent, friend, citizen). These aspects of normal living are usually classified as work, leisure and self-care.
- The use of activities as specific therapeutic media to treat dysfunctions in the performance of occupations, interactions and roles.

Solving performance problems

The occupational therapist uses a variety of techniques to assess abilities and deficits, to retrain skills and to problem solve in these occupational areas. The individuals requiring this service are frequently those who are disabled rather than dysfunctional. Once environmental constraints are removed or methods of using residual skills to best advantage have been mastered, such individuals can become independent and contributing members of society. Therapists working in the community are likely to spend much of their time in solving performance problems and adapting environments.

Application of activities as therapy

The selection of a therapeutic activity requires that a balance be achieved between the needs and interests of the patient, the personal repertoire of skills possessed by the therapist and the requirements of the model or approach within which the therapist chooses to work. Activities should be specifically selected for the individual patient with a view to a defined goal, e.g.:

- Assessing ability
- Meeting a need
- Solving a problem
- Providing experience
- Improving a skill
- Stimulating an interest
- Promoting independence
- Encouraging an interaction
- Stimulating exploration
- Providing opportunities for choice.

Activities may be used casually for recreation or as pastimes; such use is perfectly valid in the right context. This may be called diversional occupation, *but it is not occupational therapy*.

Whilst engaging the patient in remedial activities remains a central professional skill, for many therapists it may play a relatively small part in their interventions, which will be concerned more with the analysis of dysfunction in occupational areas and the consequent problem-solving actions, as described above.

Techniques of analysis, adaption and application

There are two aims for occupational analysis.

- To understand the nature of the occupation, activity or task. This is focused on the thing to be done and is necessary when selecting or adapting some aspect as therapy or trying to gain a better understanding of what the occupation, activity or task involves (occupational analysis, activity analysis, task analysis, applied analysis).
- To understand the nature of an individual's participation and performance and what it means to him. This is focused on the person as 'doer' and enables problems and needs to be understood and treatment goals to be set (performance analysis, participation analysis, analysis of meanings).

Occupational analysis

This may include: contextual evaluation of whether the occupation is work, leisure or self-care. The therapist's traditional division of occupations into work, leisure or activities of daily living must be acknowledged as artificial. In practice the edges blur. Classification is contextual – what one person regards as a chore may be a hobby for someone else. Is housework work or self-care? This method of division and particularly the currently popular concept that life should contain an appropriate balance of the three occupational areas is biased towards developed Western-style cultures and may require considerable modification in cultures where such distinctions break down. However, it remains a convenient method of analysis.

Work: Any problem which prevents an individual who wishes to work from doing so is likely to have considerable social, psychological and economic consequences. The therapist may use industrial therapy, work-related rehabilitation, adaptation of the workplace and preliminary vocational guidance and training to assist return to work. More complex vocational guidance and retraining is not within the scope of the therapist.

Leisure: Awareness of self-actualization needs and the importance of the quality of life is increasing, and a proportion of the people who are unemployed and of the growing number of retired people find it hard to cope with unstructured time and need guidance; for those who are unable to work due to a disability or illness, leisure may become crucial in giving purpose and meaning to life.

Activities of daily living (ADL): These activities range from those fundamental for survival (personal activities of daily living (PADL)) – eating, keeping warm, avoiding danger, maintaining personal hygiene and, in some settings, basic social skills – to the more complex aspects of personal self-care and independent living such as cooking, shopping and housework (domestic activities of daily living (DADL) also known in the USA as instrumental activities of daily living (IADL)).

Assessment is carried out to identify the nature and severity of the problem. A programme of practice and training is then provided in as realistic a setting as possible. Any residual disabilities which persist after a period of training are resolved by the provision of adapted equipment, environmental adaptation or assistance for the individual.

Activity analysis

This involves dissecting the activity into its component parts (tasks) and sequence, looking at its stable and situational components and evaluating its therapeutic potential.

A preliminary analysis will consider the basic content of the activity in terms of, for example:

- The kinds(s) of performance needed to achieve the activity – e.g. cognitive, motor, interpersonal (the headings used for detailed analysis will depend on the approach being used or a comprehensive analysis may be attempted)
- The degree of complexity of the activity
- The positive or negative social or cultural associations
- Whether the activity is structured or unstructured

- Defining the tasks of which the activity is composed
- Analysing the sequence of task performance and whether this is fixed or flexible
- Defining the tools, furniture, materials and environment required for completion of the activity
- Defining and taking account of safety precautions or risk factors.

Task analysis

Similarly, this involves a detailed analysis, breaking down the task into subtasks and analysing the general categories of motor, cognitive, perceptual or interactive skills required at each stage or at a particular stage. This may include an analysis of specific movements and the types of muscle action or groups of muscles used to produce these. There are two main purposes for this exercise: either to select an appropriate task to meet a therapeutic aim or objective or as a means of analysing the precise area or cause of a performance problem.

Skill analysis

Conducting a full analysis of all the skills or subskills required to perform a particular task can be complex and time consuming. A task is performed as a gestalt, and 'unpacking' the components of performance or identifying the relationships between these and causes of dysfunction is not easy. The process is normally conducted by means of close observation and the use of knowledge of anatomy, physiology, perception, cognition, learning theory and theories of human interactions. It is usual to impose some kind of structure on such an analysis. Setting norms for performance is also difficult and is the object of research; unfortunately the 'super fit' population frequently chosen for such studies renders the data inapplicable for most OT purposes. A list of headings used in skill analysis is given in Table 4.2. All these lists contain further subdivisions, which indicates the complexity of skill analysis or assessment. Although authors have

used different taxonomies, it is possible to see similarities between the three lists. These headings are also used in performance analysis to assess the levels of competence attained by the patient.

Applied analysis

This is meaningful only in relation to defined objectives and the assessed condition of the patient. Whether the therapist is selecting a single therapeutic activity or a range of options to offer the patient or is seeking to modify the activity/task to make the performance of it possible, the content of the activity/task must first be analysed and evaluated using activity analysis, and then applied to the particular situation and the needs, interests and wishes of the individual by means of applied analysis. Aspects to consider might include, for example:

- Patient's preferences and interests
- Potential for engagement of patient interest and participation
- Potential for choice or decision making
- Potential for therapeutic adaptation to meet treatment objectives
- Whether the activity is familiar to the patient – need for training or preparation in order to participate
- Evaluation of whether or not the activity will meet the specified treatment objectives.

Selection of task for use as therapy: This may include:

- Select task which offers potential to achieve the therapeutic objective. Consider motor, sensory, interactive, cognitive, symbolic, expressive factors
- Analyse task, breaking it into component parts: subtasks, skills, subskills. Decide which portions of the task have therapeutic value and require emphasis/are irrelevant or inappropriate/are to be done by the patient/should be done for the patient
- Decide need for adaptation of tools, materials: identify need for preparation.

Table 4.2   Examples of taxonomies of performance skills

Model of human occupation (Kielhofner 1995 ch 8)	Adaptation through occupation (Reed 1992 pp 124–139)	Adaptive skills (Mosey 1986 p. 42 Table 3.1)
Motor	*Sensorimotor*	*Sensory integration*
Posture	Sensory awareness	Integration of tactile subsystems
Mobility	Sensory processing	Postural and bilateral integration
Coordination	Perceptual	Praxis
Strength and effort	Motor	
Energy	Neuromuscular	
Process	*Cognitive*	*Cognitive function*
Energy	Level of arousal	Attention, memory and orientation
Knowledge	Orientation	Thought processes
Temporal organization	Attending behaviour	Levels of conceptualization
Organizing space and objects	Attention span	Intelligence
Adaptation	Recognition	Factual information
	Memory	Problem solving
	Reality testing	
	Association	
	Categorization	
	Concept formation	
	Sequencing	
	Problem solving	
	Judgement of safety	
	Generalization of learning	
	Integration of learning	
	Synthesis of learning	
	Time management	
Communication and interaction	*Psychosocial*	*Social interaction*
Physicality	Social:	Interpretation of situations
Language		Social skills
Relations	Social conduct	Structured social interplay
Information exchange	Socialization and conversation	
	Role behaviour	
	Dyadic interaction	
	Group interaction	
	Interpersonal relationships	
Social interaction	Psychological:	*Psychological function*
Acknowledging	Role identity	Dynamic states
Sending	Self concept	Intrapsychic dynamics
Timing	Locus of control	Reality testing
Coordinating	Mood	Insight
	Initiation/termination of activity	Object relations
	Coping skills	Self-concept
	Self-control	Self-discipline
	Self-efficacy	
	Self-expression	

Activity synthesis

Combining components of the activity and environment to produce a desired therapeutic outcome.

Adaptation to activity

The activity may be presented in unadapted form or may be adapted to meet treatment goals.

This is frequently tackled at the level of task adaptation since the adaptation required may differ from one stage of the activity to another. Typical adaptations are:

- *Environmental*, e.g. location, setting, milieu; press
- *Equipment*, e.g. quantity of tools/materials, adaptation to tools

- *Social*, e.g. number of people, degree of interaction
- *Physical*, e.g. position, strength, range of movement
- *Cognitive*, e.g. complexity, sequence, need for instructions
- *Emotional*, e.g. interest, meaning, self-expression
- *Temporal*, e.g. duration, repetition
- *Structural*, e.g. order of tasks, omission of non-essential tasks.

Grading

Manipulating factors required in the performance of a task or activity to meet treatment goals. Grading typically includes changes to:

- Sequence of task/components
- Size/shape of tools
- Position of tools/furniture/materials
- Quantity/specification of materials
- Speed/duration/repetition of performance
- Requirement for specific movements to perform task
- Strength required
- Perceptual components
- Cognitive components
- Simplicity/complexity
- Type of/quantity of instruction/demonstration/sample
- Context (temporal, environmental, social, cultural) of the task
- Location and content of the environment in which the task is performed
- Number of participants: requirement for interaction with others
- Degree of choice/creativity/decision taking/planning and problem solving.

Environmental analysis and adaptation

This is another area of expertise used in a way which is unique to occupational therapists.

Content analysis

Occupational therapists recognize that the environment can have an important beneficial or detrimental effect on the individual. Analysis of the content of the environment – at work, at home, at school, in an institution, out of doors, in a public place – may provide information on the causes of problems for the individual, explanations for behaviour or ideas or suggestions for therapeutic modifications.

Demand analysis

This is closely linked to content analysis and explores the psychological, cultural and social impact of the environment with reference to the effects of these factors in facilitating or inhibiting participation in occupations and activities.

The way in which environmental analysis is carried out depends on both the needs of the patient and the approach within which the therapist is working as these will alter the significance of the components which are observed.

In general terms, the occupational therapist will observe and acurately record environmental content – e.g. buildings, interiors, heat, light, sound, vibration, degree of stimulation, social or cultural significance, emotional impact – and define the environmental demand (syn. press) elements which contribute to or detract from patient performance.

There is extensive discussion in the literature of the criteria for the selection or rejection of activities for use as therapy. Enduring arguments are:

- Should OT only use purposeful, constructive activities? Are talking, thinking, imagining, relaxing, counselling, exercising, positioning, legitimate OT tools?
- How far should activities be adapted – is there a risk of 'adapting the activity out of existence'?
- The therapist often values the process above the product – but the reverse may be true of the patient. Can both be satisfied?
- How directive should the therapist be in the selection of therapeutic activities? How much choice should the patient have?

Q What is your opinion on the above questions? Make a few notes and then analyse what this indicates about your preferred model(s) and approach(es). Is your answer influenced by the nature of the client group with which you are working? Discuss your answers with others. Do you believe there are 'right' and 'wrong' answers?

Adaptation

The therapist may then alter, remove or add to elements of the environment, e.g. physical features of buildings, access, sound, colour, lighting level, temperature, decor, furniture, information content, in order to remove obstacles to performance or to enhance the opportunities for performance, learning or development.

Practical therapeutic skills

Because occupation is the foundation of intervention occupational therapists use productive, creative and technical activities as therapeutic media. This means that each therapist must also have a repertoire of practical and creative skills at a sufficient level to provide the client with safe, flexible and imaginative activities in a range of situations.

Typical skills include:

- Trade and technical skills, e.g. woodwork, metalwork, horticulture, printing, computer operation, typing, word-processing
- Craft skills, e.g. weaving, rugmaking, macrame, pottery, sewing
- Creative and expressive skills, e.g. art, collage, drama, mime, puppetry, music, dance, creative writing
- Domestic skills, e.g. cooking, budgeting, menu planning, domestic activities, DIY, garden maintenance
- Leisure skills, sport, hobbies, recreational activities, games, 'keep fit', outings.

Specialist skills and techniques

All therapists require a basic repertoire of specialist skills. Whilst these will develop with experience, basic practitioners typically have some experience in a representative range of techniques.

Examples may include abilities to:

- Make and fit orthoses
- Instruct in use of prostheses
- Assess for, provide and train in the use of wheelchairs
- Make recommendations for the provision of housing adaptations for disabled people
- Use neurodevelopmental handling, positioning and stimulation techniques (e.g. Bobath, PNF, sensorimotor techniques)
- Test and retrain perceptual-motor function
- Use behavioural modification techniques
- Conduct social skills training
- Use reminiscence and reality orientation
- Use projective techniques and media including music, art, creative writing, bibliotherapy
- Use psychodrama, role-play, guided fantasy and related techniques.

Some of these techniques will be learnt within the context of specific frames of reference for which they are appropriate. For example, projective techniques may be associated with an analytical AFR whilst Bobath technique would be used within a neurodevelopmental frame of reference.

5

LINKING THEORY WITH PRACTICE

CLINICAL REASONING

When a health care professional encounters a new client he must make sense of the case, understand and diagnose the problem and, in collaboration with the client, decide what to do. This involves high-level cognitive processing which is known as *clinical reasoning*. For some 40 years these reasoning processes have been studied in doctors, nurses and other professionals and, over the last decade, in occupational therapists.

Clinical reasoning can be defined as: the process of systematic decision making based on an identifiable professional frame of reference and utilizing both subjective and objective data accrued through appropriate assessment/ evaluation processes (Hopkins & Smith 1993).

It is important that therapists understand and reflect upon their own reasoning processes in order to become more effective practitioners. Analysis of clinical decision taking may illuminate the practice and processes of occupational therapy. Burke and De Poy (1991) write that:

An understanding of the clinical reasoning process may reveal the unique ways that occupational therapists come to assess and seek solutions to patients' problems and to delimit the scope of their practice to what is uniquely occupational therapy. Clinical reasoning addresses many of the unstated thoughts and formulations that therapists develop when they work with patients.

There are some important points in this passage: clinical reasoning involves the cognition which underlies the process of naming, framing and problem solving; secondly, and even more fundamentally, it concerns the cognitive patterns which translate the knowledge, skills and values of the therapist into action and which ensure that occupational therapists practise OT, and not some other form of intervention. Thirdly, it involves thinking which is complex, often so rapid that it seems 'intuitive', and by its very nature hard to capture and describe.

Therapists are people; they process information and make judgements and decisions like all other human beings. Secondly, they are health care professionals, they share elements of the knowledge and skills which are common to all these professions, and they think in ways which are basically similar to doctors or nurses or other professionals. Thirdly, they are occupational therapists who have a unique body of knowledge and practice which influences the conclusions they reach and the actions they take.

The OT process provides the organizing structure for practice, but as already noted it is not unique. It is the use of clinical reasoning which results in occupational therapy.

Once you have learnt to 'think like a therapist' you go on 'thinking like a therapist' and, although you may be given the same set of facts about a patient as the doctor or the nurse, the physiotherapist or the social worker, the way you describe the problems and the actions you take ought to be different. Because you have learnt the knowledge and skills of an occupational therapist, and because you understand the nature of OT and its core concerns and practices, even though you are using the same mental mechanisms as other health workers, you will think and act like an occupational therapist, and not like a doctor or a nurse.

Of course in practice the roles of various professions merge and overlap, but it is important for OT as a profession, and for its effectiveness as a therapy, that the unique focus of the profession is not submerged by multidisciplinary practice. Well-developed clinical reasoning enables the therapist to maintain this clear focus.

The study of clinical reasoning in OT is relatively recent and the terminology is still developing – indeed, in this respect, it is rather like the study of theoretical structures. It can become confusing when reading various books and papers to discover that (by now you will not be surprised!) similar terms are used by different authors to mean different things. The student needs to remember that this literature is based on a relatively small number of influential studies, mostly in America; try to see past the rather confusing terminology to the basic concepts which are being described.

Reasoning modes

There does seem to be agreement that OTs use several different reasoning modes. Mattingly and Fleming (1994) describe 'three track reasoning'. Some of these reasoning modes are similar to those identified in studies of medical reasoning and are quite well understood; other modes have been proposed as distinctly characteristic of occupational therapists.

Box 5.1 summarizes, in simplified form, the main reasoning modes which have been described to date. If you are interested in finding out more about clinical reasoning, you will need to refer to the texts listed at the end of the book.

Cognitive processes

Effective clinical reasoning depends on the use of some basic cognitive processes, so it may be helpful to summarize these.

Cognitive processes are defined as 'Mental processes of perception, memory and information processing by which the individual acquires information, makes plans and solves problems' (Atkinson et al 1993).

The phrase 'acquires information, makes plans and solves problems' is a reasonable summary of what the occupational therapist does when planning and initiating an intervention, a process in which the major part of the therapist's actions may often be 'thinking in order to do', rather than actual 'doing'.

This definition therefore highlights the main mental processes involved – perception, memory

Box 5.1 Modes of clinical reasoning

Reasoning mode	Purpose
Scientific reasoning	To understand the nature of the health condition affecting the individual, the likely consequences for activities and participation and the way in which contextual factors may change this (Schell 1998).
Diagnostic reasoning	To identify functional problems towards which occupational therapy will be directed; to make problem statements about occupational performance; to define desired outcomes, set goals and develop solutions. Diagnostic reasoning employs the four-stage model of hypothetical reasoning: cue acquisition and pattern recognition; hypothesis generation; cue evaluation; hypothesis testing (Rogers & Holm 1991).
Predictive reasoning	During predictive reasoning the therapist weighs probabilities and possibilities and attempts to predict the effects of options for intervention and to gain a picture of probable outcomes in the case in relation to various imagined scenarios (Hagedorn 1995b).
Procedural reasoning	To select solutions, procedures and actions which the therapist and/or patient may use to achieve the desired outcome or any associated objective. Procedural reasoning gives the experienced therapist rapid access to appropriate, automated patterns of action and interaction (Mattingly & Fleming 1994).
Pragmatic reasoning	In its simpler form this mode addresses the practicalities of therapy – evaluation of whether an action is feasible, and whether the context and resources in a given situation facilitate an intervention or make it inadvisable. It has also been suggested (Rogers & Holm 1991) that it also takes account of the therapist's knowledge, skill, and interests and wider organizational, sociocultural and political considerations.
Ethical reasoning	Through ethical reasoning the therapist evaluates proposed interventions in relation to the moral and ethical basis of practice, and with regard to any medico-legal considerations. There are clear guidelines on ethical practice which all therapists must follow. Ethical reasoning becomes especially important in situations where the patient is vulnerable and unable to express personal wishes or where resource limitations impose choices and priorities.
Interactive reasoning	As proposed by Mattingly & Fleming (1994), this takes place during therapeutic use of self to modify the therapist's approach in response to what the patient says or the non-verbal signals he produces. The therapist uses interactive reasoning to gain rapport, to promote trust, to motivate the patient, and to gain empathetic understanding of him as a person.
Narrative reasoning	As proposed by Mattingly & Fleming (1994) this involves the use of clinical story-telling either as an aid to understanding the patient and planning therapy or as an aid to reflective practice by analysing the informal stories which therapists tell each other when describing practice.
	Narrative reasoning has since been developed as a technique for exploring personal occupational meanings and preferences (Schell 1998).

and information processing – and the skill components of these processes. These in turn are associated with and developed through learning and experience.

The information processing model of cognition involves input, coding, storage and retrieval. Input is crucial, for if information is not attended to and coded correctly it cannot be stored or retrieved.

Information may be processed in serial form, only one source being attended to at a time, or in parallel, in which several sources of information can be dealt with simultaneously. Some forms of processing are automatic and used unconsciously, others require attention.

Pattern recognition

In order to recognize a pattern the observer must use the sequence of observe pattern → identify cues → determine pattern → relate to type. Much of the research into pattern recognition has been focused on visual perception; however, the principles can be extended to wider contexts. People tend to perceive stimuli according to factors such as proximity, similarity and closure (perceptual patterning) and impose organization on any perceived pattern in order to see it as a whole (gestalt).

Pattern recognition requires attention, the conscious focusing of perception on selected stimuli (cues) in the environment. The stimulus has to be encoded and recognized '… associated correctly with a category (or person). This is a high level process that requires learning and remembering' (Atkinson et al 1993).

Coded memories of patterns are stored in various ways as mental representations. Opinions vary as to how this is achieved; some theorists propose that information is stored in long-term memory in the form of visual or verbal representations, whereas the propositional theory of coding states that it is abstract and concerned with meanings. There is research evidence to support both theories.

The therapist uses pattern recognition continually in order to identify medical conditions or familiar problem situations or patterns of dysfunction. Patterns must be matched to those stored in memory. The memory store is searched using top-down and bottom-up strategies which enable recognition to occur. The memory is able to 'flash up' a potential match very quickly when the pattern is familiar. Pattern recognition is used during the generation of hypotheses.

So, for example, if the OT sees a patient sitting slumped in a chair, weeping, reluctant to talk or participate in activity, she may identify a potential pattern of depression. The cues acquired include posture, sad expression, lack of verbalization and lack of purposeful activity. The therapist can generate a hypothesis about the nature of the problem – 'this patient may be depressed'. However, the wise therapist will not jump from a hypothesis – an explanation which needs testing – to an assumption – a statement accepted as true for the purposes of action. The hypothesis must first be tested.

In this example the therapist might talk to the patient to see if depressive thoughts are expressed; she may talk to other staff to see what their impressions are, and she will look in the patient's case history to see if there is a diagnosis of depression.

If the pattern match continues, the therapist may decide to proceed on the assumption that the patient is depressed. But the pattern may not match; the patient may be recently bereaved, but not clinically depressed; the emotional lability, slumped posture and lack of speech could be due to a stroke or a head injury, the lack of engagement in activity to inappropriate environment or lack of meaningful opportunities for engagement. All these (and more) might be in the therapist's mind as alternative hypotheses to be tested.

Information contributing to pattern recognition may be stored in various forms: as a prototype or stereotype – a typical example of a person or object; as a schema – abstract representation of events, objects and relationships in the real world; as a frame – a data structure representing a stereotypic situation; as cognitive maps; or as templates, which enable the whole pattern to be matched at once.

Experts can develop a store of many thousands of patterns as 'chunks' in which both the pattern and the action it requires are stored together and appropriate responses appear rapidly as soon as the pattern is detected.

Productions, scripts and procedures

Actions or cognitive strategies may be stored as procedures (sequences of actions) which can be encoded as production systems or 'mini-procedures'. Productions link to form sets which together form the behaviour for a larger task. A production may be stored as a simple formula 'if X happens, then do Y', possibly modified by some other circumstance, 'provided that…'

Actions may also be stored in the form of a script, a stereotypic sequence of actions appropriate to a situation – once the situation is identified the actions can be smoothly sequenced according to the script.

There is some evidence that therapists acquire scripts for some of their familiar actions and situations, e.g. a script for a first interview or a particular form of assessment (Hagedorn 1995b).

PROBLEM SOLVING: COMBINING COGNITIVE PROCESSES

Recognizing patterns and associating these with possible actions and consequences is part of what the brain does when problem solving. Problem solving is a basic human skill and one which is important in therapy; as previously noted, the OT process is in fact a version of the problem-solving process.

Although we tend to speak of 'problem solving' this is rather misleading. We need to consider the process in three parts: *problem naming, problem framing* and *problem solving.*

Problem naming, framing and solving

Naming the problem means 'saying what it is'. The therapist needs to help his client to define what is unsatisfactory in the current situation and what, ideally, the client would like the situation to be.

Framing the problem means choosing to put an interpretation on how to describe and deal with it. For example, 'not going out of the house' could be seen as a problem of mobility, but it might equally be a problem of access (steps in the way), motivation (doesn't want to go out), social isolation (no one to visit) or the result of a specific diagnosis such as agoraphobia. Each interpretation would lead the therapist to take a different approach and a different course of action to resolve the problem. In some cases more than one frame is applicable, but care must be taken to see that solutions remain compatible.

Once naming and framing have been completed – at least in preliminary form – the therapist and patient can jointly agree on priorities and goals. Only then can the therapist work with the client to design the means of achieving the desired outcome. The therapist may be equipped with a mental store of solutions, but he can only provide an appropriate solution in the context of an individual and his or her needs.

The problem may turn out to be one familiar to the therapist or it may be something novel, in which case the therapist must think out a new solution on the basis of his knowledge and experience or enable the client to do this for herself – true 'problem solving'.

It may be apparent to the therapist that there is a problem, but the client may not wish to recognize or deal with this. In fact, getting the client to accept that there is a problem can *be* the problem.

Conversely, the client may be seen by others as having or causing problems whilst the therapist may be able to see that the problem does not lie with the patient, but rather with the physical or social environment or the nature of the problem task.

It is possible to identify that, although a problem may exist, intervention is unnecessary, ineffective or not beneficial. Some problems are incapable of solution, and many require some compromise or adaptation to be made.

Complex problems may require analysis from a variety of perspectives and theoretical frameworks, each of which may provide a different explanation or course of action. Unravelling such complex situations is very challenging. The skill of finding alternative ways of 'naming and framing' problems is closely linked to the use of models and frames of reference, as will be described later.

Cognitive aspects of problem solving

Problem solving can be conceptualized as taking place in a mental problem space, a 'box' into which all the available information is put and in which the problem solver manipulates the elements of the problem. 'It contains states of knowledge about the problem. Both the initial situation and the desired situation are represented as elements of this space ... problem solving is always a matter of search' (Newell in Johnson-Laird & Wason 1977).

The problem solver must identify the problem and then find a means of moving from the initial state to a state where the goal is satisfied by means of an operator – some appropriate strategy or action. A heuristic – 'a strategy that can be applied to a variety of problems that usually, but not always, yields a correct solution' (Atkinson et al 1993) – may be used as an operator. Sometimes problems may be solved by insight, in which the solution is suddenly presented without intervening stages of development.

A familiar solution may become a mental set which may limit problem solving if the problem solver becomes hooked into one particular solution which worked before and cannot change this set when faced with a different but superficially similar problem. A client can become caught in this trap and become unable to see a way out of her difficulty for herself. A therapist must also beware of becoming dependent on familiar solutions to the exclusion of others.

When the problem is complex or unfamiliar, the mind generates a series of 'what if' hypotheses and previously learnt rules which seem applicable and tests these against the desired state. At this stage production of many possible strategies is useful. Good problem solvers are very flexible, have well-developed lateral (divergent) thinking and use strategies such as 'brainstorming' to produce a multitude of creative and novel solutions.

Evaluation and selection of solutions is another key stage in the process: effectiveness may not be the only criterion, e.g. one may need to consider acceptability to the client or others, time, resources, effort, cost and practicality.

The stages in the OT process will now be described in more detail.

Collecting information

The key to problem solution is gathering sufficient information about the situation. This may occupy much of the time spent on the problem and will involve reference to many sources – the client, other people or professionals, casenotes, textbooks and so forth. Once it is possible to identify accurately what the problem is, a solution is frequently obvious. Attempting to solve a problem which is inadequately understood or where too many assumptions have been made is seldom successful.

Having too much data is often a bigger difficulty than having too little. The ability to select the relevant from the irrelevant comes with experience. Expert judgement and knowledge may be required. The creation of expert systems – computer data bases and diagnostic programmes aimed at helping with clinical problem solving – is a recent development to assist doctors and other professionals. So far there have been few attempts to create expert systems for use by therapists (Arnold & Penn 1990). Information

processing is now an important separate branch of knowledge, both in computers and in cognitive psychology.

Problem identification

If the therapist has seen a similar problem before, he can rapidly identify it. Cues are recognized and matched to memories of previous clients and there is a rapid shift from understanding the problem to deciding what could be done about it.

Some situations are unfamiliar or more complex and need more analysis. This involves providing answers to questions such as: what is the problem? Is there more than one? Which is the most significant? Which should be tackled first? The apparent or obvious problem may be a symptom rather than the real cause of the difficulty. Action may turn out to be inadvisable or impossible.

Some people are uncomfortable with the word 'problem'. In this context it simply means defining the needs of the client which are to be the areas for intervention by the occupational therapist (diagnostic reasoning). Putting it another way, the 'problem' is the therapist's initial lack of understanding of the individual and her situation; until sufficient data is gathered, and goals set, action cannot be taken by either the therapist or the client.

The logical sequence in which problems are tackled is also important. Effort can be wasted by dealing with subsidiary issues which would be resolved by solution of the root cause. On the other hand, the client may not be ready to tackle 'the big one' but may be able to gain confidence by succeeding with something smaller. Whittling away the peripheral problems with easy solutions can also help to build confidence in the problem-solving process and will help to reduce the big problem to a more manageable size.

Identification of the desired outcome

Identification of the problem – the 'undesired state' – must bring with it a clear specification of the 'desired state'. This is not the same as a solution, which is the method whereby that state may be achieved and which may sometimes be far more difficult to identify. The desired outcome may be clear, but the route to it hard to find.

Much depends on the client's perceptions of her needs. Defining the desired outcome requires negotiation between therapist and client. Goals should never be imposed.

Often there is only one desired outcome but sometimes there may be alternatives, which can be evaluated for comparative benefits, put in priority order, discarded or kept in reserve as a viable alternative if the first choice proves unattainable.

Goal setting is an essential prerequisite for therapy or intervention, and it is often necessary to define goals in terms of timescale – immediate or longer term – and to subdivide them into objectives. An objective should contain a clear statement of what is to be achieved and some means of measuring the outcome.

Solution development, evaluation and selection

The human brain is uniquely geared to be effective at problem solving. At a low level it can do this so rapidly that it appears intuitive, although this is actually based on fast processing of previous knowledge and experience together with insightful connective jumps between pieces of information.

The more experienced the therapist, the bigger his mental stock of available solutions and actions will be. Students, however, lack this resource and will inevitably take longer to sort out what to do.

Again, possible actions need to be checked out with the patient, and her approval must be gained. Actions which a client clearly rejects, however beneficial, cannot be carried out.

Development of an action plan

The *action plan* specifies the stages by which the solution will be implemented and the desired state achieved. It should also clarify who is responsible for doing what. Although the plan should not become too rigid, clarity in specifying the goal, timescale and method of testing success

or failure is helpful and assists outcome measurement.

An action plan may relate to action by the therapist, but it may equally well define action to be taken by the patient or others.

Implementation

The plan is put into action and the process and results are recorded. It is important to keep checking that the plan is moving towards the target. The therapist must keep in mind any service standards or quality statements to ensure that practice meets these requirements. All interventions must be well documented.

Evaluation of results

The effectiveness of the action is measured against progress towards the previously agreed outcome. Once that is achieved, intervention ceases or moves to another problem. Compromises may be necessary. Action may uncover previously unsuspected problems which need to be dealt with. Action which is ineffective must be changed. Was the solution wrong? Was the problem incorrectly defined in the first place? Is the problem insoluble or the gain not worth prolonged effort? Answers to these questions usually require a return circuit round the problem-solving process, gathering more information and redefining the problem.

Problem-based recording systems

Problem solving is often associated with problem-based systems of recording, particularly problem-oriented medical records (POMR) (Weed 1968, 1969) and the SOAP system.

Problem-oriented medical records

Using this system, the problems experienced by the client are identified and listed. They may be categorized under headings according to a standardized system and may be allocated numbers. Once listed, problems are prioritized and may be divided into short-term and long-term goals. An intervention plan is designed and implemented for selected goals. It is useful to separate the elements of the plan which will involve the client's direct participation from the things which the therapist (or others) will do. All references to the intervention and subsequent progress in resolving the problem refer to it by number. When the problem is resolved, it is removed from the list and subsequent problems may be tackled (King's Fund Centre 1988).

Putting this recording system into practice requires some effort, but once set up it does aid teamwork and concentrates efforts on practical issues by identifying the action to be taken and the most appropriate person to take it, and facilitating review of progress.

SOAP

SOAP is a method of problem identification and solution. SOAP stands for:

Subjective
Objective
Assessment (or Analysis)
Planning.

First, the client's subjective view of her situation is obtained and recorded, together with the subjective views of any other people involved.

Following this, the therapist will identify some likely problem areas and investigate these objectively by formal observation and assessments.

The results of these procedures will then be analysed in order to decide what the problem(s) might be. At this stage it may become clear that the client's subjective view differs from the objective assessment of the therapist or from the subjective views of significant others and this mismatch may in fact constitute the problem. Once a problem list has been composed it is possible to decide on action.

The planning stage involves selecting priorities, goal setting, generating possible solutions and selecting the preferred one, and putting the plan into action, as described earlier in this chapter.

Although SOAP does not contain another stage, it is implicit that the success of the plan is monitored and reviewed and action modified accordingly. The number of problems solved at the end of the intervention can be used as an outcome measure.

When using this system, all actions by the therapist are recorded with the key letters S,O,A,P. For example, an interview with the patient would be under S; an observation of the occurrence of a particular difficulty would be under O, together with the number of the problem observed; a case conference might be A or P; the treatment plan would be P.

Using this system does take practice and requires a certain mental discipline, but once proficiency is attained it can greatly speed up and simplify the process of keeping case records, as well as making goal setting and planning more precise. It also offers the advantage of a measurable outcome which is of considerable value in implementing quality assurance audits and producing evidence of the results of therapy.

There can be difficulties in fitting actions or occurrences into the SOAP format, and the system should not be allowed to get in the way of good recording. Some forms of problem-based systems include a 'strengths and needs' assessment of the individual – Individual Programme Planning is an example – so that strengths can be built on as part of the problem-solving process. This also avoids the risk of a rather negative problem list which may result in the patient being viewed as a 'problem'.

POMR and SOAP may be linked to a key worker system, where an individual is given the responsibility of managing a case and coordinating effective therapy.

HOW MODELS AND FRAMES OF REFERENCE AFFECT THE OT PROCESS

So far we have been examining the cognitive processes which take place during problem naming, framing and solving. You now need to understand how a model or frame of reference can be used to inform or structure this process.

The key to the way this works is the point at which the selection of a theoretical structure is made. If it is selected *before* the therapist meets the client and begins data collection it can function as a conceptual lens (Kielhofner 1992) affecting and limiting subsequent actions. If it is selected later in the process, once the nature of the problem is becoming apparent, it acts as a tool for the job, ensuring that intervention is appropriate and coherent.

I refer to selection of an approach before intervention commences as being theory driven; here the form of assessment, content of clinical reasoning and process of naming and framing the problem are directed by the selected theory.

Selection of an approach after the problem is named is referred to as being process driven because the process of naming and framing the problem automatically suggests which approach will be most applicable.

In both cases the therapist remains conscious of the core principles and processes of OT: to lose sight of these might result in the therapist drifting off line into the selection of approaches and actions which, while valid in themselves, are not relevant to the practice of OT.

Theory-driven practice

If you imagine putting on a pair of coloured spectacles you know that what you see will be subtly altered. The view will be tinted in some way. If in addition the spectacles magnify what you are looking at or restrict the field of view so that you can see only part of it, the effect on your perceptions will be even more marked.

If you select an approach (put on the spectacles) before you have even met your client, you will view her and her problems through that filter. You may decide to be theory driven for philosophical or practical reasons.

For example, you may decide that the Canadian Occupational Performance Model is an ideal expression of OT practice. You then use the language of the model, its conceptual constructs and the assessment (Canadian Occupational Performance Measure (COPM) – see Section 4) which has been developed for use within it. You do not normally use any other initial approach (although you may legitimately select one at a later stage, once the problem has been named and framed within the model).

On the other hand, it may be obvious, because you work in a specialized area, that only one applied frame of reference is relevant. If you work on an orthopaedic unit you will probably base your intervention on a biomechanical approach; if you work with neurological disorders a neurodevelopmental approach will be more useful; if your clients have psychosocial needs you may decide to use a group work approach. This is a simple matter of common sense; it would plainly be inappropriate to treat a psychosocial disorder using a specific physical approach (Fig. 5.1).

Process-driven practice

If you work in the community or in any area where you have a wide range of clients, the theory-driven pattern may be too restrictive. You need to retain the option to use a number of approaches, depending on the nature of the problem which you and the client have identified as most significant.

You use the OT process to work with the client to name the problem and decide how best to frame it. You then select which of the available approaches to use as a tool and generate solutions or plan actions within that approach.

Of course, you need to choose the right tool for the task. Sometimes there is a wide choice, and at others a narrow one. If you need to knock in a nail you automatically pick a hammer, not a screwdriver. To drill a hole you can choose from an electric drill, hand-drill, brace and bit, bradawl or auger. This may seem confusing, if you are not a carpenter to whom the choice will be obvious. Similarly, the selection of the right approach becomes easier when you have expertise as a therapist (Fig. 5.2).

Process-driven practice can be depicted as a circular version of the OT process, with escape

Q Before reading further, spend some time considering the advantages and disadvantages of these two ways of using theory.

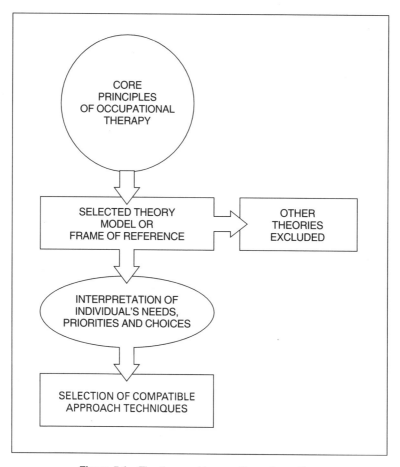

Figure 5.1 The theory-driven pattern of practice.

routes and subsidiary pathways for exploration and definition of issues (Fig. 5.3).

Alternatively you might use the DARE structure explained in Section 3.

Theory or process driven?

If you did the analytical exercise you will probably have concluded that both patterns have advantages and disadvantages. For example, being theory driven provides you with a coherent and consistent basis for practice and eliminates unnecessary deliberation. It promotes the development of expertise within a defined field. However, it could be restrictive, with the therapist trying to fit the client to the theory come what may, and selection of a very narrow

approach could ultimately reduce the therapist's abilities.

The process-driven approach has flexibility, but demands a highly versatile and competent therapist who is confident in clinical reasoning. Some approaches require considerable expertise and should not be used unless there is an experienced supervisor available. Being process driven is not the same as being casually eclectic, mixing and matching theories and techniques as they come to mind; care must still be taken to be consistent within the selected approach and, when combining approaches, to check that they are compatible.

These two patterns of practice are suited to different situations. It is quite possible to move

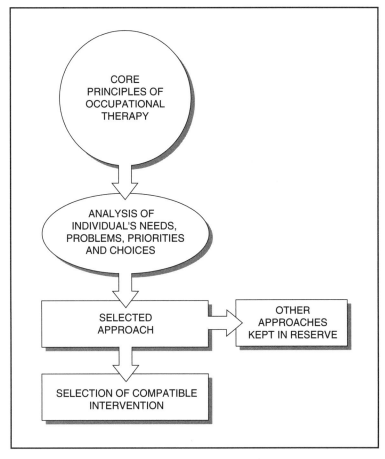

Figure 5.2   The process-driven pattern of practice.

from being theory driven to being process driven if required and indeed this does happen within some PEOP models.

Spot the approach

When you enter a new situation it may not always be clear which approach is in use. It may be there for situational or historic reasons which are unstated. The users may not have conceptualized what they are doing in terms of 'using a model'. There may be several different approaches being used by different individuals or team members.

A little detective work is required in order to decide whether a model or AFR is being used. The clues include:

- Attitudes: are there any obvious attitudes or values which underpin action?
- Language: what kind of words are being used to describe the individual and the OT process? Are these mainly medical or more informal? Are you dealing with a patient or a client? Are there any key words in use which indicate a theoretical basis for action?
- Assessment procedures: what is being assessed? Is this a narrow area of occupational performance or skill or is it broadly based? Which assessment tools and methods are in use? Is assessment conducted by the therapist or by the client? Are any outcome measures in use?

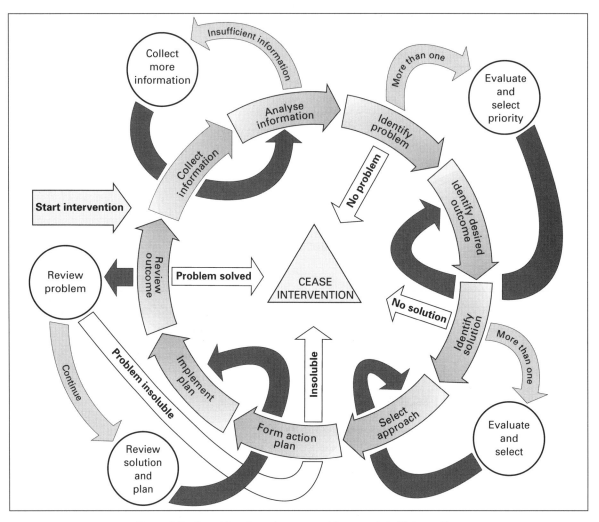

Figure 5.3   A problem-based, process-driven model of intervention.

What kind of intervention is being provided? Does this appear to be process driven and problem related or theory driven?

ARE THEORETICAL STRUCTURES REALLY NECESSARY?

It is possible to know a great deal about OT theory and to remain an indifferent therapist: theoretical knowledge alone does not guarantee competence in practical application. On the other hand a therapist whose practical competencies are enhanced and informed by a sound theoretical understanding will certainly be a better

practitioner than the one who ignores theory and does what seems common sense at the time.

There is, however, a catch: studies on the way therapists think tend to indicate that there is a progression in clinical reasoning from being a novice practitioner who 'does it by the book' to becoming an expert practitioner who has 'thrown the book away' (see Schell 1998).

A paradox of practice, due to the way in which reasoning occurs, is that the more experienced and expert you become, the more theory becomes embedded into practice, and 'knowing' is expressed as 'doing', until it can actually become very hard to unpick it again. Thus it may be difficult for an expert therapist to explain to the student 'why I did that' or to track back to the underlying theory and principles.

The antidote to this problem is to develop the skills of the reflective practitioner who regularly takes time out to stand back from his practice, analyse what he is doing and challenge himself to justify it and seek improvements.

Can one learn how to reason more effectively?

It might seem that the answer ought to be 'yes' – that if you understand more about how your mind and memory operate, and about the uses of logic, the laws of probability and formal analytical information processing techniques, you should become a more effective reasoner. An understanding of cognitive psychology, especially in relation to information processing, is certainly useful.

Unfortunately, the evidence from studies of structured attempts to teach medical students more effective forms of reasoning, or better problem solving, have not been very conclusive. In general, such training makes less difference than one might expect, although the more closely it is linked to actual practice – e.g. realistic role-plays and simulations of real problems or patients – the better.

It may be that there is simply no substitute for rich and varied experience in real clinical situations. However, there is some evidence that considering such experience in an active, critical and reflective manner does help to develop good reasoning skills over a period of time.

Developing a personal model

Each therapist is an individual with a unique experience of life both personal and professional. You have your own personal world, your own meanings and associations. Even if you went to the same training college as someone else you cannot guarantee that your experiences there, or what you remember, will be the same as the other person's. As you practise as a therapist you will build on your basic training in an individual way. Whilst OT is recognizably OT in most

countries, if you speak to any ten individual therapists you are likely to get ten different versions of OT.

It has, therefore, been suggested that each therapist develops what is in effect a personal version of OT – a 'personal model' (or paradigm) (Kortman 1994, Tornebohm 1991).

Having reviewed the personal nature of clinical reasoning it becomes easy to see how this happens. The occupational therapist has her own set of values, attitudes and opinions about OT theory (a personal version of the paradigm). The stored memories of lectures, courses, books and papers, the solutions, productions, scripts and procedures, and the images of past patients will all contribute to this personal model.

At one level this is exciting and challenging; many of the applied frames of reference and OT models presented in this book probably originated from the personal model of the author. OT needs the impetus of personal model building in order to develop its theory and practice. It needs therapists who can capture, analyse and communicate their personal practice for the benefit of others.

At another level there needs to be a note of caution. The therapist does need to review her personal model at intervals to check that it has not deviated from currently accepted practice or become stale or out of date. That new idea, that exciting technique may be very good and very interesting – *but is it OT?* A personal model may pick up unconnected material, and needs periodic spring-cleaning. One must return to descriptions of the OT paradigm, and use these to check one's personal version for consistency.

The practitioner must also guard against becoming over-automated, a situation particularly likely to occur when treating very familiar types of cases where reasoning is so smoothed out and habitual that the formula is used as a substitute for original thought.

Reflecting on personal practice and discussing it with others, using supervision actively, and keeping up to date with the professional literature are important ways of keeping on track.

Reflective practice

There are many techniques which aid reflective practice: keeping a personal diary of ideas, feelings and experiences; discussing cases with others; telling therapeutic 'stories' and learning from them. It is also useful to try more structured analytical techniques: for example trying to recapture all the elements of a situation, to relive it to see what the hidden agenda might have been, and then to alter the script, to rehearse different actions and reactions, testing them against what actually happened.

However it is achieved, it is the quality, depth and efficacy of clinical reasoning which differentiate the novice from the competent practitioner, and the competent practitioner from the expert (Slater & Cohn 1991, Schell 1998).

Frames of reference

6

Primary frames of reference

As described in Chapter 3, there are two types of frames of reference: *primary*, which contains 'borrowed knowledge' derived from sources external to OT, and *applied*, a synthesis and interpretation of that knowledge for use in OT which I have called 'the OT version'. To avoid repetition I will use the abbreviation PFR to indicate primary frames of reference and AFR to indicate applied ones. (The distinction is useful but in practice it may be simplest to use 'frame of reference' as an umbrella term.)

A primary frame of reference contains theories and knowledge which have evolved within one of the basic sciences. When knowledge is complex it may be divided into branches or described according to a particular perspective or set of theories. Primary frames of reference which are relevant to OT are those which contain information about how a human being functions in daily life and propose explanations to account for dysfunction.

Occupational therapy has been informed by theories from many different primary frames of reference; however, these have not all resulted in applied frames of reference. In some cases, just one or two ideas have filtered into OT, whilst in other cases a whole set of theory and practice has been adopted and adapted. Three important primary frames of reference which have resulted in 'OT versions' are:

- The physiological frame of reference
- The psychological frame of reference
- The educational frame of reference.

Because occupational therapists deal with human performance, during which biological and psychological processes must be integrated, they frequently mix elements from primary frames of reference when formulating an applied frame of reference. For an AFR to be effective, however, this synthesis must only include compatible elements. It is important, therefore, to remain true to whatever AFR one has selected and to be cautious about using more than one at the same time for the same patient, unless they share a closely related theoretical basis.

THE PHYSIOLOGICAL PRIMARY FRAME OF REFERENCE

The physiological PFR is associated with the biomedical model. It is concerned with the ability of the body to maintain homeostasis in response to internal and external changes (Fig. 6.1). Electrochemical processes control actions, reactions and the individual's ability to respond to and learn from the environment. Performance depends on genetic potential and the integrity and interactions of all body systems, principally the musculoskeletal system,

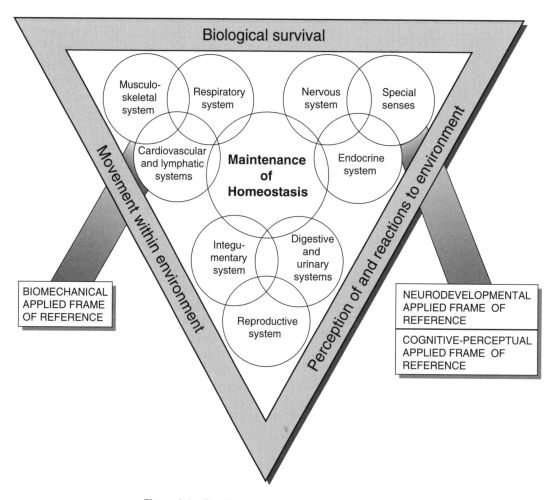

Figure 6.1 Physiological primary frame of reference.

cardiovascular system, neurological system, endocrine system and the special senses.

The internal mechanisms of homeostasis are of background interest to the therapist, but not the main concern. In order to maintain homeostasis the individual must drink, eat, avoid danger, move around in the environment, keep sufficiently warm and so forth. Whilst these actions are partly controlled by automatic bodily processes, they also require active participation by the individual to ensure that the necessities of survival are obtained. The person needs to:

- Move and perform functional actions within the environment
- Perceive, interpret and react adaptively to environmental stimuli.

It is these aspects which concern the therapist. Thus, this PFR has given rise to various applied frames of reference (AFR) (with associated approaches) of which the following are the most important:

- The biomechanical AFR (concerned with functional movement)
- The neurodevelopmental AFR (concerned with development or re-education of motor control)
- The cognitive perceptual AFR (concerned with the way we perceive and interpret our surroundings).

In order to understand the basis of functional movement, occupational therapists need a good foundation knowledge of human anatomy, physiology and kinesiology, and a detailed understanding of neurophysiology and development.

THE PSYCHOLOGICAL PRIMARY FRAME OF REFERENCE

Psychology deals with the scientific study of behaviour and mental processes. As psychology has evolved during the last century various theories have become influential in their turn.

Psychology began by being closely linked to neurophysiology, then moved into studying behaviour, human development, psychological aspects of learning and cognition. The development of personal identity and personality, human roles and relationships and the behaviour of people in groups have also been studied.

Atkinson et al (1993) describe distinct psychological perspectives:

- Biological (the neurobiological basis of behaviour and perception)
- Behavioural (learnt responses to environmental stimuli)
- Cognitive (study of mental processes of reasoning and learning)
- Psychoanalytic (study of unconscious processes)
- Phenomenological (concerned with subjective inner experiences).

Psychology has given birth to a variety of specialities, e.g. experimental, educational, industrial, environmental, evolutionary, cognitive, social and clinical.

All the schools of psychology have been influential in OT in different ways at different times. It has to be admitted that psychology is prone to 'fashions' as each new and attractive theory is proposed and gains supporters.

During the 1980s, cognitive psychology, which deals with cognitive processes such as memory, information processing and problem solving, has been influential. Social psychology, defined as 'the scientific field that seeks to understand the nature and causes of human behaviour in social situations' (Baron & Byrne 1987), has also been very influential.

During the 1990s humanistic, client-centred approaches gained prominence.

An understanding of a range of psychological theories is essential if the therapist is to assess and identify the individual's difficulties in perception, memory, learning and performance, and therefore to construct more effective ways of presenting information or improving skills (Fig. 6.2). It is also important to understand the influence of culture and other people and to appreciate that each person creates a personal world of meanings, symbols and memories.

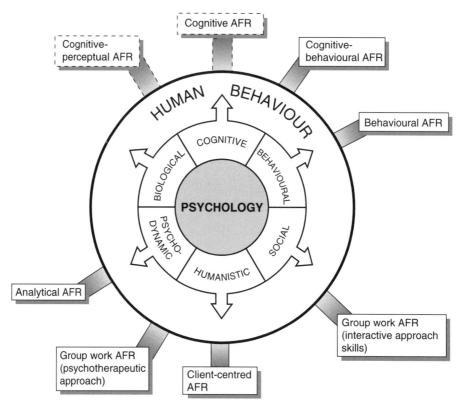

Figure 6.2   Psychological primary frame of reference.

Psychological theories abound concerning the ways in which mental mechanisms and perceptions of self consciously or unconsciously affect human emotions and behaviour.

Traditional psychoanalytical theories and, later, psychotherapeutic theories have been developed into a range of therapies for the treatment of mental health disorders and cognitive dysfunction. Those which have been adapted for use in OT are described in Chapter 8. These include:

- Cognitive-behavioural
- Cognitive
- Analytical
- Humanistic and client centred.

THE EDUCATIONAL PRIMARY FRAME OF REFERENCE

Psychology deals with human behaviour, much of which is learnt (Fig. 6.3). It is

therefore inevitable that many theories concerning the mechanisms and processes of human learning have evolved. This aspect of psychology constitutes a large field of knowledge. These ideas have been so influential in OT that they merit consideration as a separate PFR.

Education, as will be discussed in Section 3, is an important process of change. Through participation in education people are enabled to learn new things, acquire new skills and develop culturally appropriate attitudes and values. Knowledge of learning theories and models of education enables the therapist to develop a repertoire of educative strategies and skills to suit the wide range of learners and learning environments which she encounters.

Educational theorists are interested in the nature of knowledge (*epistemology*). They propose learning theories derived from various

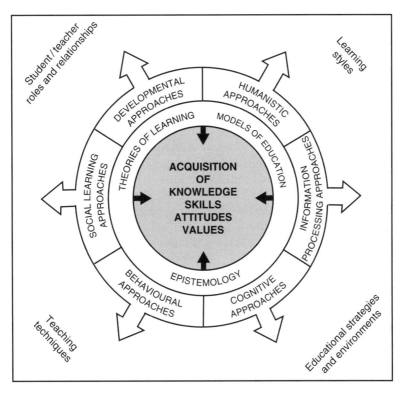

Figure 6.3 Educational primary frame of reference.

distinct perspectives (behavioural, developmental, cognitive, information processing, social and humanistic), study learning styles and the roles and relationships of student and teacher, and explore educational practice.

Applied frames of reference and approaches originating from learning theories are used for clients with physical and/or psychosocial dysfunctions. They include:

- The behavioural AFR
- The cognitive AFR
- The cognitive-perceptual AFR (compensatory and remedial approaches)
- The biomechanical AFR (activities of daily living and compensatory approaches)
- The interactive skills (group learning) approach
- The student-centred learning approach.

In addition, therapists use numerous teaching and problem-based learning techniques, all of which can be traced back to educational practices and theories.

OUTCOME MEASURES AND THE QUESTION OF EFFECTIVENESS

Outcome measures

An *outcome measure* is simply a tool whereby the results of intervention can be measured, quantified or evaluated.

An outcome measure is used within the context of a treatment plan to enable comparisons to be made between the situation at the start of intervention and that at the end, in relation to a stated objective.

Many OT assessment tools and techniques can be used as outcome measures. The basic principles which apply to any form of assessment – validity, reliability, replicability – apply with even more force when the assessment is to be used as an outcome measure. The results must be dependable and accurate or they are of little use.

This is less of a problem when there is something which *can* objectively be measured. Unfortunately, especially in settings where a client-centred approach is in use, this may not be the case. The question of how far subjective ratings of outcome are valid is a matter of dispute.

The range and quality of outcome measures available for use within each frame of reference are very variable. Where assessments have been developed for use within an AFR these have been listed. In other cases only general guidance is possible.

The question of effectiveness

If an intervention works in the sense of successfully treating a health condition or producing measurable change in a previously specified aspect of human function, it may be said to be effective. Evaluation of effectiveness is based on firm evidence, derived from research.

Clinical effectiveness is associated with, but distinct from, questions of cost effectiveness and the effective and efficient use of resources. For example, an intervention which takes six months to achieve results might be clinically effective, but might not be cost effective or an efficient use of resources. Use of effective but very costly therapies (such as very expensive drugs) may produce serious ethical dilemmas.

In the case of OT it is far from easy to prove that a specific intervention works. To do so the therapist must undertake research, with all the implications of time, cost, practicalities and the usual problems of designing a valid study.

There is a traditional, hierarchical view of the degree of value which should be attributed to findings from various forms of research. The strongest evidence is provided by *meta-analysis* in which many similar controlled studies can be compared and the results of the intervention can be proved to be successful. After that the most reliable form of study is an experimental controlled trial.

Various forms of quasi-experimental studies come next and finally descriptive studies, which are not highly regarded from the point of view of evidence. To date, although the amount of research in occupational therapy is increasing, the majority of evidence of effectiveness rests on descriptive studies. This is particularly so in mental health settings (Craik et al 1998). The necessity for improving the quality of evidence for effectiveness in OT has been recognized for some time.

It is, however, a mistake to limit the search for evidence to studies from within the OT profession, important though these are. Evidence can often be obtained from other sources. These may include reports of basic research into human physiological or psychological function, medical studies and studies of applied techniques in psychology, psychotherapy, nursing, physiotherapy or remedial education.

Literature reviews, systematic evaluation of research over a period of time in a specific area and meta-analysis of comparable case studies can all be valuable.

Even when reliable research evidence is absent a systematic and critical review of descriptive studies may prove useful. If one descriptive study claims a successful result it may legitimately be dismissed as unconvincing. If 30 descriptive studies of similar type can be assembled and rigorously evaluated, and all show similar positive results, the evidence begins to be more impressive. This type of exercise may then lead on to research to validate practice.

With so many approaches to deal with it is not practical to attempt a detailed appraisal of evidence for each one. Where such evidence is readily available I have cited some key references. Where it is not, I have included some general comments about the nature of the evidence and the degree to which the approach is, or is not, rated as effective.

Developing evidence of effectiveness is a key challenge facing occupational therapists in the next decade.

Recommended reading

There are a number of textbooks on theoretical aspects of OT and many standard texts giving descriptions of occupational therapy.

To avoid continued repetition throughout this Section these references have been included as a separate list in Recommended Reading. (Supplementary references are listed together under References). These books will be cited when a chapter contains particularly relevant material, but the reader can refer to the more general topics for supporting information or details relating to a particular client group.

In the following chapters some additional specific references will be given; readers who wish to study a particular approach in detail will need to refer to journals and other sources.

7

Applied frames of reference for physical dysfunction

INTRODUCTION

Occupational therapy in a physical hospital setting

The occupational therapist who specializes in the treatment of physical dysfunction frequently works in a traditional clinical setting within a hospital. She is typically a member of a rehabilitation team and is inevitably influenced by the biomedical model which is still predominant, especially during acute phases of treatment.

As the patient recovers and moves towards discharge the occupational therapist has an important bridging function. It is the OT who is best placed to move both the patient and the team in the direction of the social model of rehabilitation, which is a necessary prerequisite for successful discharge. The dependent patient in care becomes the independent client moving back into the community.

This change of focus can be difficult and even contentious: once acute care is ended the overwhelming need of the system is that the patient should be moved on as quickly as possible so that a new patient can be admitted. The therapist may be in the position of simultaneously trying to facilitate discharge, whilst acting as an advocate of the client's wishes, ensuring recognition of the need to keep the client in hospital until suitable social support and environmental adaptations can be made.

Health providers and managers are only slowly recognizing that hospital care needs to be structured to permit this transition, especially in the case of older people. Attempting to avoid the issues or to short-circuit the end of the rehabilitation process in order to speed discharge, whilst expedient in the short term, creates longer term problems.

The applied frames of reference described in this section have been developed within this context, and are applicable for different health conditions and at different points in the process of rehabilitation.

Other settings

Therapists also work in day hospitals, special clinics and in the community. The applied frames of reference in this chapter may be applicable here, but some need adaptation for use within the social model of disability, especially when used in the community.

SPECIALIST OT TECHNIQUES

Advances in our understanding of both neuroanatomy and the physiology of muscles, joints and the cardiovascular system are continuous. The therapist needs to discard outdated techniques and develop new ones in line with these advances.

It is noticeable that many of the references cited in support of these AFRs date from the 1980s. In the field of health care any information about human function, health conditions or therapeutic techniques which is more than 10 years old should be regarded with critical caution. Whilst some techniques are tried and tested and still in use because they work, others may have been superseded by new developments. There is a need to evaluate the results of therapy in order to justify the continued use of remedial techniques.

All of the AFRs require the use of specific competencies and some require additional training in specialized techniques. It is impossible, in these brief summaries, to do more than outline the theoretical basis and main focus of each approach. For these reasons it is essential to read widely, and to refer to the most recent sources of information when seeking to improve or develop practice.

THE BIOMECHANICAL APPLIED FRAME OF REFERENCE

The biomechanical AFR is used almost exclusively in the context of the process of physical rehabilitation. The connection is so close that the two are often confused, but the rehabilitation process is a much larger entity than the biomechanical AFR, which is just one of the AFRs which can be used to provide a framework for rehabilitation.

The 'bio' part of the title is based on kinesiology, which combines neuromuscular physiology and musculoskeletal anatomy. The 'mechanics' part indicates that it is also based on 'mechanical' laws, e.g. leverage, gravity, friction and resistance. In this AFR the therapist focuses on 'the body as a machine', usually working to improve one or more of 'the four Ss' – suppleness, strength, stability and stamina – and through this to improve function. Physical exercise, isotonic or isometric, is used to increase the strength and bulk of muscles and to improve stamina and work tolerance. Repetitive exercise is also used to increase or restore the range of movement at a joint.

Primary assumptions
- The application of a graded programme of exercise based on kinesiological principles will restore normal or near normal function.
- Biomechanical principles can be used to design orthoses, prostheses, assistive devices, mobility equipment and adaptations to equipment or the physical environment.
- 'Practice makes perfect'; repeated training improves performance.

To improve function one needs to practise and to work at the upper edge of current abilities. In a typical training or retraining programme the individual is required to work as close to his functional limits as possible, without undue fatigue, and the goal posts are continually moved as improvement occurs. Grading of the elements in the exercise programme, e.g. adding assistance or resistance, altering range, speed, duration and repetition, is often a crucial part of the therapist's role.

The biomechanical AFR has several approaches which may be used separately or at different stages in the treatment programme. Those commonly described include: the graded activities approach, the activities of daily living (ADL) approach, and the compensatory approach (Fig. 7.1).

The graded activities approach uses activities for remedial purposes, not necessarily because the person wants or needs to engage in them in his daily life. Activities may include craft techniques, DIY, sports, games and so forth. Many accounts of the biomechanical AFR are limited to this approach, transferring the others I have listed to 'rehabilitation'.

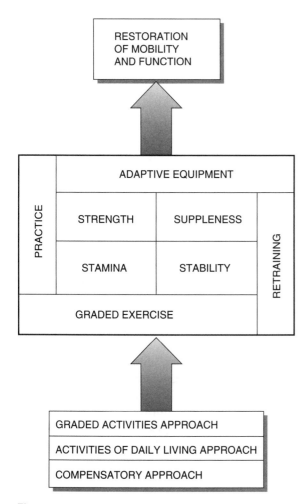

Figure 7.1 Biomechanical applied frame of reference.

In this approach the performance of an activity is used to produce specific effects; e.g. to promote defined movements, to exercise specific muscle groups or to work for extended tolerance of standing, sitting or walking.

Thorough physical assessment and measurement of function is an essential precursor to therapy. Precise measurements must be made to set a baseline from which subsequent improvement can be assessed. Measurements can include: joint range (using a goniometer), muscle power, length of time a movement or activity can be sustained, speed, number of repetitions, distance or any other precisely quantifiable factor. The selected factor must be reassessed at regular intervals in order to monitor progress and set new targets.

In order for this approach to be effective, elements in the performance must be controlled and graded with precision. This requires an imaginative and ingenious attitude on the part of the therapist, which in former times led to the use of complex adaptive apparatus, pulley circuits and the like. The use of productive activities in this way involves thought and preparation, and unless correctly used and monitored, the activity may be too generalized in effect to be useful.

It is almost inevitable that patient choice in the selection of an activity will be limited by the constraints of meeting specific physical objectives, and the product must often be subordinated to the process. This approach has been criticized as overly directive and mechanistic; it has also, ironically, been criticized as insufficiently precise. This, together with the reaction against 'craft work' and the desire to appear technologically advanced, has resulted in the use of stereotyped non-productive activities (such as remedial 'games') purely for their exercise value, and not for any intrinsic interest or end product. This trend was very noticeable during the mid 1970s, but it is now decreasing.

There is currently a renewed interest in the specific remedial use of activities as it is once more appreciated that the combined psychological and physical benefits of constructive, practical or creative activities may outweigh the disadvantages of any lack of precision in physical application.

Some interesting adaptations to computers have recently been produced, together with equipment using surface electrodes to translate specific muscle contraction into switching of electric apparatus. This is sometimes used in connection with biofeedback techniques.

The accelerated pace of recovery from trauma due to improved medical and surgical techniques during the past two decades has rendered rehabilitation unnecessary in some cases and has generally resulted in much shorter hospitalization, which has left little time for graded activity programmes to be implemented. The graded activities approach is therefore mainly used to treat individuals with more serious injuries or conditions requiring longer term treatment, which is often undertaken on an out-patient basis.

There are some individuals who just cannot relate to this approach; it is my personal view that patients whose needs are better met by exercise than activity, or who actually prefer exercises, should be referred to a physiotherapist.

The activities of daily living (ADL) approach is concerned with the movement components of functional activity. It uses biomechanical principles to improve the individual's ability to do personal or domestic activities of daily living. A basic assumption of this approach is 'practice makes perfect' – that by repeated practice, by continually challenging the individual to do a little more, praising achievements and consolidating gains by continued use of the regained skill, function will improve.

The compensatory approach is concerned with enabling people to make up for residual disability by the use of orthoses, prostheses, aids to daily living or home adaptations. This approach may come in quite early in an intervention, when the patient's abilities are limited and aids are therefore necessary. In this situation it may be possible to phase out the use of aids as recovery takes place. Alternatively, the compensatory approach may follow on from the ADL or graded activities approach, solving residual problems as the patient prepares to return home or go back to work.

This approach may also involve training in new skills, and requires a good deal of planning,

> **Q** Where do you stand on the question of the use of activities for specific physical treatment? How far should activities be adapted? Is adaptation effective? Is it too time-consuming? Should OTs use non-productive 'activities'? How do patients react to this form of therapy? Discuss these points with some colleagues: you may well get a wide range of firmly held opinions.

problem solving and lateral thinking on the part of both patient and therapist. The approach may be quite mechanistic, merely looking at assistive devices, but in a more adaptive form other compensatory changes may be needed, involving attitudinal changes and adoption of techniques such as time management, energy conservation, joint protection, pacing of activities and lifestyle planning.

In the community the compensatory approach is much used, since getting the home environment right for a disabled individual can make a major contribution to personal independence.

Outcome measures: The patient is expected to show measurable improvement in specified physical movements or in performance skills. Assessments need to be quantifiable and specific.

A wide range of standard assessments of physical function can be used.

Effectiveness: There are numerous studies of effectiveness in physical rehabilitation, but the majority do not come from within OT literature. The therapist must therefore be prepared to search widely to extract evidence to support the particular interventions or treatments she intends to use in relation to a specified type of health condition or trauma.

Effectiveness of interventions to improve function in activities of daily living may be more difficult to demonstrate, but such interventions are widely accepted as valuable.

Advantages and disadvantages: Biomechanical techniques are well researched and can be shown to produce improvement in physical function. Because improving functional ability is the chief goal and results are relatively rapid, the patient can see positive benefits as treatment progresses and is motivated to continue. Residual disabilities can be overcome by aids and orthoses.

Because treatment in the graded activities approach has to be very specific to produce results, patient choice in the selection of activities may be restricted: there is a danger that programmes may become stereotyped. Activity programmes take time to set up and prepare and are impractical where treatment time is limited. An overly physical bias may result in wider social environmental or psychological problems being ignored.

THE NEURODEVELOPMENTAL APPLIED FRAME OF REFERENCE

This is an umbrella term used to describe a range of theories concerning the way in which human movement and control develops over time.

There is always a time-lag between making discoveries through research and translating these into remedial techniques. This makes it difficult to provide a concise summary of the neurodevelopmental AFR.

Neurology is a challenging specialism which requires the therapist to have a good grasp of current theories and also some expertise in specific techniques. It is also important to be aware of the theoretical basis of treatment being provided by other members of the rehabilitation team, especially physiotherapists, to ensure that OT intervention is compatible.

There are numerous neurological conditions affecting adults and children. These arise from a variety of congenital and acquired health conditions and as a result of trauma. These conditions require different approaches. One cannot take a 'one size fits all' attitude to selecting an approach.

Neurodevelopmental approaches often originated in the treatment of children, and have been adapted subsequently for use with adults following a stroke or head injury.

Clients with spinal cord lesions, demyelinating diseases or other degenerative disorders have different problems and may need a combination of approaches.

Primary assumptions: As indicated in Fig. 7.2, this AFR is based on the following assumptions.

- Development of motor control is a prerequisite for the development of skilled movement.

- Development depends on the integrity of the nervous system and the musculoskeletal system and the ability of these systems to work together to produce intentional, coordinated responses.
- This interaction is further modified by feedback from the environment and opportunities available within it.
- Development of motor control and the acquisition of basic skills follows a definable sequence over time.
- Skill components are refined by practice and integrated to form patterns of skilled performances.
- An individual can only perform at his or her developmental level; it is not possible to develop advanced skills until foundation skills have been mastered and integrated into the repertoire. Stages of development cannot be jumped or missed.

Traditional neurodevelopmental approaches

Traditional approaches commonly used by therapists during the 1980s and early 1990s have been derived from the work of theorists (not necessarily OTs) during the 1960s, 1970s and 1980s. These include Rood, Bobath, Brunnstrom, Knott and Voss, and Peto.

Their view of motor control was hierarchical. In simplified form, the theory was that there was direct feedback between sensory input and motor output. If you stimulate sensory feedback you promote movement. Positioning and placing of joints and stretching of muscles in specific ways would promote normal sensations and inhibit abnormal patterns. A developmental sequence in which movements were acquired was also proposed; the individual must roll, crawl and sit before being able to stand, step and walk.

Bobath approach

This bilateral approach to the treatment of hemiplegia or spasticity utilizes positioning, weightbearing, reflex inhibition and sensory facilitation. It can be adapted for use with OT

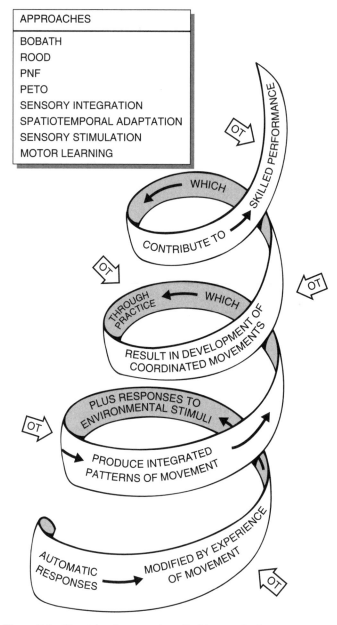

APPROACHES

BOBATH
ROOD
PNF
PETO
SENSORY INTEGRATION
SPATIOTEMPORAL ADAPTATION
SENSORY STIMULATION
MOTOR LEARNING

Figure 7.2 Neurodevelopmental applied frame of reference.

activities more readily than some other techniques (Bobath 1990) and is widely used by occupational therapists.

Basic principles include:

- Positioning the patient in a manner which will inhibit the development of abnormal reflexes and synergies and reduce abnormal muscle tone, enabling the patient to relearn normal movement patterns

- Facilitating correct movement by positioning, correct handling, use of sensory stimulation and of key control points on the body

- Working through a developmental sequence – lying, 'all-fours', trunk control,

sitting, standing, weight transfer, stepping, walking
- Involving both sides of the body in all activities. Use of activities which *promote*: crossing the midline with the arm; diagonal patterns of arm use; special bilateral grip; weightbearing through affected side; trunk rotation; and which *avoid*: flexor patterns in the upper limb and extensor patterns in the lower limb; stimulation of associated reactions.

PNF approach

The technique uses positioning and diagonal patterns of movement in developmental sequence and emphasizes sensory input, visual cues and verbal commands to produce maximum input. Sensory input stimulates and facilitates motor output. This approach is less adaptable for use in OT, except as an adjunct to therapy, but some general principles are transferable.

Conductive education approach (Peto)

This highly structured and formal system mainly used with children (although some work has been done with adults) is based on a planned, intensive programme aimed at achieving goals for each individual following a blend of cognitive and neurodevelopmental principles (Macdonald 1990). The therapist acts as a conductor planning tasks, facilitating movement, and using formalized verbalization to assist actions. The patient also says what he is doing at each stage as he does it. Personal control and responsibility are emphasized; rhythm is used to promote and initiate movement. Conductive education is currently attracting considerable interest and is used by physiotherapists, but it is not as yet widely used by British occupational therapists. It requires special training. Some therapists have incorporated the concept of patient verbalization as an adjunct to other therapy.

Rood approach

This uses similar principles to sensory integration and PNF but emphasizes tactile stimulation (brushing; icing; tapping; pressure, and stretch reflexes). Rood is both an OT and a physiotherapist but the technique is more related to PT than OT. Occupational therapists tend to use it as a precursor to other therapy.

Sensory integration approach (Ayres, King)

In the treatment of children with developmental difficulties, and children or adults with psychiatric disorders or mental handicap, the emphasis is on the capacity of the individual to perceive and react correctly to people and the environment. Recognizing the strong link between sensory input and motor output, the therapist may use sensorimotor activity to stimulate perception and proprioception, thus raising the general level of activity where this is retarded.

In this approach development is depicted as a spiral in which the individual gradually moves upwards, having consolidated gains at each level. The importance of the integration and interpretation of all sensory inputs, and the necessity of promoting integrated sensory stimulation to develop or restore function, are stressed. The link between sensory input, cortical organization and personal appreciation of the use of adaptive skills is important.

Activity (such as play) using touch, vibration, sound, smell, colour, is geared to stimulation at subcortical level, with particular attention to vestibular and proprioceptive input. This technique was developed by Ayres for use with children and neurologically damaged adults.

Another version of the technique has been used in a psychiatric setting following the work by King with schizophrenics; she advocated the use of activities which increase and promote vestibular stimulation, bilateral integration and the integration of primitive postural reflexes to overcome synaptic barriers and promote normal body image, posture, righting reactions and reflexes.

Both approaches are complex and require considerable study, so it is essential to read the longer descriptions given in the reading list (Reed 1984).

Spatiotemporal adaptation approach

This is similar in some ways to the sensory integration approach. It is also designed for use with children. One of its main assumptions is that interaction with the environment shapes development, which is again seen as a spiral process. Occupation is seen as a context which provides purpose and motivation which help to promote and shape motor performance. Again, this is a complex approach which requires careful study and practice.

Sensory stimulation

This approach is used to provide richly stimulating input to one or more senses. To achieve this, colour, scents, sound, texture, movement, vibration, flashing lights, and different types of touch are used to promote a reaction. The quality of the reaction will depend on whether the combination of sensory inputs produces a relaxation response or stimulates alertness and attention. This approach is most often used with individuals who have a severe learning disability or brain damage. The Snoezelan environment is an example of sensory stimulation.

Advantages and disadvantages: When used correctly and intensively these therapies claim to produce good results, particularly in preventing the development of abnormal patterns of movement and deformity following neurological damage.

Unless used intensively, skilfully and correctly by all members of the treatment team, results are likely to be disappointing. Special training is required to use most techniques effectively. Working neurodevelopmentally is time-consuming and functional recovery in the brain-damaged adult, e.g. walking, may be delayed with consequent frustration for the patient. The techniques are less suitable for use with very elderly patients. Extreme highly intensive versions of some techniques, particularly when applied to children, are still very controversial.

Recent neurodevelopmental approaches

There have been many recent advances in our understanding of the physiology and neurochemistry of the brain and the nervous system and the complex mechanisms which interpret sensation and produce movement. Some of these developments have challenged thinking which has been current in neurological rehabilitation settings for the past 10 or 15 years.

The 'cause and effect' view of the operation of the nervous system is now seen as oversimplified. The nervous system is not hard wired but plastic; control and learning may originate at various levels. Motor control is now viewed as highly complex, involving many body systems in an interactive, global dialogue. Skill development does not just depend on these interactions but also on precise forms of feedback from the environment and the added factor of personal motivation. These ideas are only slowly filtering into OT practice.

As is usual at a time of transition the result is a considerable variation in practice, some therapists' techniques being based on older AFRs and others on more recent ones. For example, Wilsdon (1996) describes the traditional neurodevelopmental approaches and Pulaski (1998) appears to favour a traditional rehabilitation approach based on functional activity. However in the same book, other authors describe more recent approaches such as motor control.

Dunn (1997) summarizes neuroscience from an OT perspective, and Poole (1997) compares the assumptions of traditional rehabilitation treatments with contemporary models and describes new frames of reference including views of motor learning influenced by systems theory and the ecological approach. She describes the Motor Relearning Programme (MRP) proposed by Carr and Shepherd (1987) and a task-oriented model of neurological facilitation (Hovak 1991). Giuffrida (1998) also describes 'motor learning' which she sees as 'an emerging frame of reference for occupational performance'.

Primary assumptions

- Both neurological and non-neurological factors affecting performance should be considered.
- Skilled movements are developed through structured task performance.
- Performance may be improved by controlled and directed feedback, specific forms and duration of practice, and attention to task selection.

A demand for competence

All neurodevelopmental approaches demand a high level of competence from the practitioner. They involve detailed knowledge of neurophysiology and musculoskeletal anatomy. Specific techniques require skill and must be practised extensively before use.

In several instances the techniques were originated by physiotherapists and are not readily related to activity-based therapy, being more commonly used as an adjunct to or precursor of this.

It is unfortunate that, in the past, occupational therapists have sometimes been tempted to use these techniques at a rather low level of skill. Whilst it is not necessary to be an expert it is necessary to be competent. Incorrect use of neurodevelopmental techniques at best is ineffective and at worst might be damaging.

Therapists who wish to use these techniques are urged to do so initially under supervision from an experienced practitioner.

In the absence of such expertise the therapist can use a different approach, e.g. dealing with performance problems using compensatory techniques such as environmental or task adaptation.

Outcome measures: Specific approaches generate their own outcome measures. The validity of these is variable. The therapist should seek those which are appropriate and well researched.

Effectiveness: The question of comparative effectiveness of these techniques has not been settled. Proponents make good cases for most of the traditional techniques. It has been argued, however, that the improvements which patients make may be due as much to the close and facilitative relationship which develops between an expert therapist and the individual, the intensive nature of the therapy and the expectation of improvement as to the specific therapy.

In the USA and UK there are national guidelines for the treatment of stroke, which should be referred to (US Department of Health and Human Services 1995, Intercollegiate Working Party for Stroke 2000).

As already noted, there has been much recent research, and this may provide new evidence. There is a need for more research into the outcomes of OT interventions within these approaches.

INCOMPATIBLE AFRS

You should by now have realized that the approaches of the biomechanical and neurodevelopmental AFRs are incompatible. Although both AFRs are soundly based on physiology, each uses a distinct knowledge base, and the resultant techniques are mutually exclusive.

Unless this is clearly understood there is room for a good deal of confusion and, consequently, ineffective therapy.

As a generalization, the biomechanical AFR is reductionist in philosophy and is used in the rehabilitation of musculoskeletal or peripheral neurological injury, whilst the neurodevelopmental AFR is more holistic and is used in the treatment of trauma or developmental delay/regression affecting the sensorimotor systems in children or adults.

The most significant opposing principles of the two AFRs are summarized in Box. 7.1. This does, however, represent a simplification and it must be remembered that application will vary in accordance with the needs of individuals with specific conditions.

Box 7.1   Incompatible AFRs

Neurodevelopmental AFR (Bobath approach)	**Biomechanical AFR (graded activities approach)**
Work first for control and pattern of gross movements.	Work first for functional use. May promote fine movements.
Always work from proximal to distal.	May work from distal to proximal.
In the upper limb use extensor/abductor patterns. Promote grip last. Avoid stimulation of flexor surfaces.	In the upper limb work for flexion and functional use – promote grip early. May use stimulation of flexor surfaces.
In the lower limb work against extensor thrust and adductor patterns.	In the lower limb promote knee and hip extension and stability of knee and ankle.
Delay walking and standing until developmentally ready.	Stand/walk as early as possible.
Grade therapy according to developmental stages: work within limits of current level until ability to progress is established.	Grade therapy according to progress: work at or just beyond limits of current capacity.
Use orthoses and external supports with discretion and as a last resort.	Use orthoses as routine.
Emphasize treatment of whole body to achieve symmetry.	Emphasize treatment of affected part.
Emphasize sensory integration and proprioception.	Emphasize functional and protective sensation.
Do not encourage compensation by one part of the body for lost function in another.	Encourage compensation for lost function by using a different body part.

THE COGNITIVE-PERCEPTUAL APPLIED FRAME OF REFERENCE

Perception is a cognitive process which involves the interpretation and identification of sensory information within the brain. If damage occurs to the brain, the ability to interpret such information can be affected. This may result in difficulties in performance due to incorrect assumptions about the environment leading to faulty motor control. Knowledge concerning the environment, and also knowledge of patterns of movement which enable appropriate responses to be made when information is received, are also stored in the brain and can be damaged.

The cognitive-perceptual AFR is concerned with these 'hidden' mental processes which enable a person to: know where he is; recognize objects or people; move around within a defined space; carry out purposeful movement; learn; remember; use logic; problem solve; cope with use of concrete and abstract language.

Primary assumptions
- Perception and cognition are essential prerequisites for functional performance. If recognition of incoming information is defective or an appropriate response cannot

be organized, the individual will be unable to perform functional activities.
- It may be possible to improve perceptual or cognitive deficits by intensive practice and retraining.
- It may be possible to assist a person to compensate for perceptual or cognitive deficits.

Perceptual deficits include many different disorders. Two important groups are the agnosias and the apraxias. It is important to distinguish between a perceptual or cognitive deficit which originates from damage to the parts of the brain which recognize, store and interpret information, and deficits due to damage to the peripheral organs which receive or transmit that information. In agnosias and apraxias there is no physical damage to these organs.

An agnosia (i.e. absence of knowing) is an inability to use information or recognize a concept which was previously familiar. For example, inability to count objects or to tell the time, inability to recognize a part of one's own body.

An apraxia (i.e. absence of skill) is an inability to perform a previously known skill, although the instruction to do so is understood and the physical ability to do so is intact. This could include getting dressed, manipulating objects, writing or pattern making.

There are other deficits such as visual field problems and body image problems which also cause functional difficulties.

The cognitive perceptual AFR has three approaches: diagnostic, remedial and compensatory (Fig. 7.3).

The diagnostic approach

The *diagnostic approach* requires a very good understanding of neuroscience and the complex mechanisms of perception. The therapist uses performance tests and special assessments to identify the type and degree of perceptual deficit. An experienced therapist can often make a diagnosis from observing functional performance just as well as by using tests; deficits in test performance do not always correlate with functional difficulties, but may support a diagnosis.

Having decided what the problem is, the therapist can then decide whether to attempt treatment to improve the ability or intervention to compensate for the loss. Even if it proves impossible to improve function, it is important to

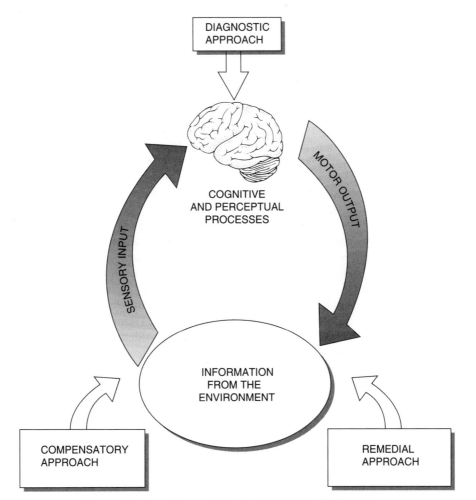

Figure 7.3   Cognitive-perceptual applied frame of reference.

understand the extent of the deficit, which can sometimes be covered by a good social manner or natural adaptability. A perceptual deficit may seriously affect skills such as driving even though motor function is intact.

Perceptual deficits can be hard to diagnose, especially when several are present at once. They may occur in adults with brain damage from a variety of causes who also have other problems which may make diagnosis difficult. Perceptual deficits also occur in children and may be associated with developmental delay. These usually respond to treatment more readily than deficits caused by trauma.

The remedial approach

The remedial approach involves training or retraining the perceptual skill by intensive practice, but success in the case of brain-damaged adults may be only partial. It is debatable whether improvement is due to the practice or simply to spontaneous recovery as the acute phase following trauma subsides. One theory which explains recovery deals with 'brain plasticity', i.e. the capacity of the brain to compensate for damage by relearning, and by using unaffected spare capacity to make up for that which has been lost. Another theory deals with the ability to generalize a skill learnt in one context to another, e.g. by practising patterns in order to improve writing or copying designs in blocks in order to improve spatial awareness. Computers have recently been used to assist in perceptual training.

One of the difficulties in treating severe forms of perceptual deficit is that the patient may be unaware of the problem because the damaged area of the brain has no means of communicating the extent of the damage to the intact areas. There is a gap in a visual field or a problem in using a part of the body, but the person simply fails to realize the nature and extent of the deficit. It is plainly very difficult to teach someone to compensate for a deficit which, for him, does not exist. It is equally difficult for new learning to occur if perception or memory is affected.

The compensatory approach

The compensatory approach involves teaching the individual to use other perceptual abilities or providing additional cues and prompts in the environment which promote perception. Such cues may include: positioning of objects; breaking down tasks into stages; presentation of information in small quantities; verbal cues; social cues or prompts; use of distinctive colours or shapes to help in identification of objects (see also cognitive AFR, Chapter 8).

Outcome measures: Many therapists continue to use informal and unstandardized assessments of perceptual function. Whilst these can provide useful indicators of dysfunction they are not good outcome measures.

There are numerous standardized tests of cognitive and perceptual function and when the assessment needs to be deficit-specific these should be used wherever possible (see, e.g., tests listed in Duchek & Abreu 1997; Golisz & Toglia 1998).

In addition to specific cognitive tests, various functional measures may be used.

Effectiveness: It can be important to identify 'hidden' perceptual deficits as these may have a marked effect on the individual's performance and may, at times, place him at risk if not noticed (e.g. allowing a person with a large visual field deficit to continue driving). However, whether retraining is effective in actually removing the deficit or in compensating for it is less clear.

Once again, the therapist needs to search the literature to find whether forms of cognitive/perceptual retraining produce measurable change. This question is complicated by the problems which affect much research in this area: learning is a complex process. In the case of acquired brain damage a cognitive or perceptual problem may resolve with time, along with other dysfunctions, without specific intervention (however, intervention may speed this process).

It seems likely that effectiveness will depend on skilled use of retraining techniques and very precise forms of prompting, cueing and feedback.

Advantages and disadvantages: The cognitive AFR deals with an area of function which is frequently ignored by other specialists. Suitable practice or other intervention may improve function.

The tests used require experience for accurate interpretation and may take time to administer. It may be possible to identify a problem, but not possible to do much to improve the situation.

8

Applied frames of reference for psychosocial dysfunction

INTRODUCTION

As noted in the last chapter, applied frames of reference evolve over time. Ideas about the origin of mental problems and techniques for dealing with them have been proposed by theorists whose assumptions come from very different perspectives.

Earlier views of human behaviour were deterministic. More recent ideas have explored cognition, and holistic concepts related to self-image and individuality. There is still a debate over the degree to which human behaviour depends on 'nature': that is, genetic predisposition and other biological factors; or 'nurture': that is, the effects of the social and physical environment. Because human behaviour is learnt many of the AFRs originate from or use theories of learning.

We have seen that in physical rehabilitation the biomedical model has been challenged by the social model. A similar process has occurred in mental health settings. The use of the term 'mental health' in place of 'mental illness' is a symbol of this attitudinal shift. However, there remains a tension between the pharmacotherapeutic approach of 'a pill for the patient's problem' and the more psychotherapeutic client-centred approaches.

The environment of practice has also changed. Much of the infrastructure of hospital care which formerly supported the provision of occupational therapy for people with long-term needs has been dismantled. Work in the community poses new challenges.

Partly for these reasons therapists in mental health have moved away from traditional forms of therapy based on occupation, and have been placed under some pressure to become generic, doing very similar things to psychologists, psychotherapists or mental health nurses. In a survey (Craik et al 1998) two-thirds of OT respondants working in mental health settings in the UK indicated that they were involved with non-occupational therapy tasks.

The authors of this study conclude that there is a need to ensure that occupational therapists in mental health are using their core skills, and also a need to conduct more research in this field in order to provide evidence of effectiveness.

Under the influence of recent client-centred occupational performance models there has been a conscious attempt to return to an occupational focus, using activities with individuals and groups.

This means that the more deterministic approaches and also those based primarily on verbal techniques are seen as less appropriate. These approaches are included because they have been influential in the past and remain valid in specific circumstances.

Occupational therapists work with people in the context of their performance problems. Although they may, in certain settings, be interested in the underlying psychodynamics, therapists are practical people who need pragmatic approaches to assist their clients.

Cognitive approaches use recent research into learning and memory to improve information processing and task performance.

The cognitive behavioural approach is now well established and there is good evidence of effectiveness in conditions such as depression and anxiety. This approach fits well with occupational therapy, as it recognizes the links between thoughts, feelings and behaviours. These can be considered in the context of tasks and the modifying influence of the social or physical environment of performance.

Group work based on activities may provide practice of social skills or can be used to stimulate group exploration of ideas and feelings. The benefits of being absorbed in shared

---

BOX 8.1 AFRs and approaches described in this chapter	
AFR	**Approach**
Behavioural	Behavioural modification
Cognitive	Multicontext treatment approach (Toglia)
	Integrative functional approach (Duchek)
Cognitive	Cognitive behavioural
Analytical	Freudian and Neo-Freudian approaches
	Projective techniques approach
Group work	Psychotherapeutic group approaches
	Interactive skills approach
Client-centred	Person-centred ethical practice
	Client-directed approach
	Therapeutic alliance
	Student-centred educational approach

activity are being rediscovered (Clark et al, 1998).

The humanistic client-centred approach is now widely used in the process of goal setting and intervention. Much of the recent literature in OT emphasizes the importance of being client centred.

The approaches in this chapter are presented in outline form. The challenge of adapting approaches developed by other professions for use in OT without losing the essential occupational focus remains.

BEHAVIOURAL AFR

Behaviourism is primarily a theory of learning. This has developed from the original research into stimulus response learning by Pavlov, Thorndike and Watson, followed by the work on operant conditioning by Skinner and many others. Research is concentrated on proposing explanations of observable human behaviour in terms of interaction with the environment. The environment provides stimuli to which the individual responds. The individual is able to appreciate the outcome of the response by means of feedback. Responses which are rewarded or are useful to the individual in satisfying drives are continued and become part of the behav-ioural repertoire. Those which are unsuccessful, or which achieve unpleasant results, are discontinued.

Hard line behaviourists believe that the individual has little choice in deciding how to behave, being 'programmed' to react through conditioning derived from past experience. All interior motivators such as emotions and thoughts are discounted either as products of behaviour or as internal, unobservable, and therefore incapable of objective study.

Bandura (1977a,b) extended the concept of operant conditioning and recognized that the individual does not need to experience the reinforcement personally, but may learn by observing the results of the behaviour of others, a process called *modelling* which has important implications for therapy.

Other researchers have moved away from the extreme behaviourist position and have tended to include some elements of cognitive theory, particularly aspects of the information processing theories of memory, learning and decision making.

Few occupational therapists apply the behavioural frame of reference in strict and unadapted form, but behavioural theories have been influential in both education and therapy, and are used in behavioural modification and desensitization programmes, and in skill training and programmed learning.

A feature of all such programmes is the breaking down of tasks into simple component parts and sequences and the use of very clear statements of objectives, goals and methods of instruction, and of schedules of reinforcement, designed to meet the learning needs of the individual (Fig. 8.1).

Primary assumptions

- An individual can only be studied in terms of her observable behaviour. All actions performed by the individual are regarded as behaviour; this includes language.
- Behaviour occurs in response to stimuli which promote or decrease it.
- All behaviour is learnt. Behaviour can be unlearnt (extinguished) as well as learnt.
- Learning occurs in response to reinforcement which is either provided extrinsically by the environment or intrinsically by the behaviour. Intermittent schedules of reinforcement are the most effective.

- A positive reinforcer must be carefully selected to be appropriate to the individual and must be correctly and consistently used.
- Behaviour can be reduced to a simple sequence of responses: these can be taught separately if required or chained in sequence. Complex sequences combine to produce 'molar behaviour', the response of the whole organism.
- Learning programmes should be designed to meet the exact requirements of the individual.

Terminology: Behaviourism has a distinct language which must be acquired to work comfortably within the approach. Frequently used terms include: classical conditioning; operant conditioning; stimulus-response (SR) conditioning; deconditioning; extinction; positive/negative reinforcement; schedules of reinforcement; reward/punishment; time out; modelling; shaping; cueing; training; behavioural contract; behaviour modification; goal planning; behavioural objectives.

Behaviour modification approach

As an OT technique it is most frequently used with people who have learning disabilities, to teach part skills as a means of building up more complex behaviours or to remove behaviours which are damaging to the person or others, an approach known as *behaviour modification*. Behavioural principles are also used in psychiatry but, apart from desensitization of phobias or anxiety, it is now more usual to employ a cognitive behavioural approach in this field.

A typical behaviour modification programme might involve:

- Settting a precise behavioural objective for the patient to achieve: this involves detailed task analysis so that a portion of behaviour can be isolated and taught
- Deciding on a positive reinforcer or reward to be used following successful performance, e.g. food or drink, an enjoyable activity, praise, affection, a privilege. (At this point a

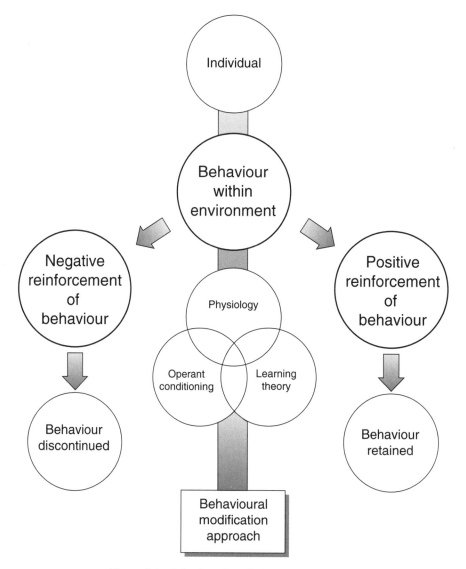

Figure 8.1   Behavioural applied frame of reference.

behavioural contract specifying both the desired behaviour and the reward may be drawn up between client and therapist)

• Providing opportunities for the behaviour to occur, prompting, shaping and cueing the behaviour if necessary

• Providing the reward (consistently/intermittently) when the behaviour (or at first, a close approximation to it) is achieved

• Gradually withdrawing or reducing the frequency of the reward once the behaviour has become an established part of the repertoire.

The keys to the successful use of this approach are breaking down the task, defining a clear objective, finding a reinforcer which is acceptable and effective, and, above all, a very consistent implementation of the programme by everyone involved with the patient.

Writing behavioural objectives

Writing clear behavioural objectives is an essential therapeutic skill which is often used even when not employing a behaviour modification approach. It is also a skill which is not always carried out with sufficient precision. This is mainly a matter of practice. An objective must contain both the specification of the performance and criteria by which successful completion can be measured. It is usually formed as follows:

- Person (student/client)
- Precise performance (define what is to be done)
- Conditions (when, where, how often, how long, with/without specified form of help).

For example, the student (person) will point to the carpal bones on the skeleton and will correctly name each one (precise performance) at the first attempt and without reference to notes (conditions).

Outcome measures: Because of the highly structured nature of this approach there are clear outcome measures, usually phrased as behavioural objectives. The degree to which these have been achieved can readily be evaluated.

Effectiveness: Behavioural modification is a long-established technique with good evidence

of effectiveness, although the therapist will need to refer to literature from psychology and psychiatry to find it.

However, behavioural modification in its pure form is now used less frequently than forms of cognitive behavioural therapy.

Advantages and disadvantages: Precise objectives are set, and achievement of objectives is measurable in performance terms. The associated techniques are of particular use for individuals who have moderate or severe learning difficulties, challenging behaviours or behavioural disturbances, and for people with fears originating from situational conditioning. Learning does not have to depend on patient motivation or cooperation. Teaching can be tailored to individual needs. Specific skills and sub-skills can be learnt in small stages. Behaviours can be unlearnt.

Although basic behavioural theory is often used, effective application of behavioural techniques is time-consuming and must be done with great precision and expertise by all concerned; this normally requires additional training. Incorrectly applied behaviour modification is at best useless and at worst damaging. Each objective must be very carefully phrased, specifying the behaviour and the conditions under which it will be performed: if this is done 'fuzzily', therapy may be ineffective and measurement of success of dubious validity. Learning may not generalize and may fade once the reinforcement is withdrawn. The reductionist approach ignores emotional and cognitive explanations of behaviour. An overly strict application of positive/negative reinforcement, particularly if there is any element of punishment or deprivation, carries ethical implications and should be avoided.

COGNITIVE AFR

Cognitive psychology is concerned with the information-processing capacities of the brain. These may be studied from various perspectives, e.g. identifying the precise areas of the brain which operate during various forms of cognitive processing, making comparisons between human

---

If you would like to practise writing behavioural objectives, try producing some for this client

Jenny is a 16-year-old girl with severe learning difficulties. She has been referred with the aim of 'improve independence in feeding'. When you visit her at lunch time you observe that she at first makes no attempt to feed herself. She is able to grasp a spoon when it is placed in her hand and rather messily tries to get some food onto it. Once she has the food in her mouth she immediately tries to get some more onto the spoon and into her mouth without leaving time for chewing and swallowing, and consequently spits out food or chokes and becomes very frustrated. She abandons her attempts at eating after a few minutes. She is very fond of music and also likes to touch a favourite cuddly toy bear.
1 Write some clear behavioural objectives for the first stage of your treatment.
2 Which would you tackle first? Would you work towards this in stages? If so, how might you write specific objectives for this?

processing and that of artificial intelligence in computers or studying the cognitive processes which underpin learning and memory, and evaluating ways in which specific intervention can improve these functions.

These aspects can be further related to developmental, educational or adaptive processes.

In OT the cognitive AFR is most frequently used when dealing with acquired cognitive dysfunction, such as memory, attention or learning deficits occurring after head injury or as a result of degenerative brain conditions such as dementia, long-term psychosis or as a consequence of drug abuse. It also has application in learning disabilities.

Key assumptions

Cognition depends on the ability to perceive, interpret, store, relate and retrieve information (Fig. 8.2). This process is complex, involving several parts of the brain, many cognitive skill components and different forms of memory.

Basic cognitive processes are governed and evaluated by metacognitive processes which play a key part in organizing effective performance. Cognitive skills and processes are intricately connected with the use of language. Although the model of cognitive function is now well understood much remains to be discovered about the actual physiological mechanisms involved in encoding, storing and recalling information.

Research indicates that people employ various cognitive strategies at different levels of performance. Some of these operate automatically without the individual being aware of them, whilst others may be consciously employed. If the individual has poor cognitive strategies, both learning and the capacity to act will be impaired. This may be due to a failure to develop good strategies to begin with or to subsequent damage to the brain which affects the capacity to use such strategies.

It seems that a key component in developing good strategies is that the individual gets accurate and immediate feedback to indicate which strategies are effective, and is therefore able to monitor the results of his mental processing.

If performance is to be useful it must be freely transferable from one situation to another and

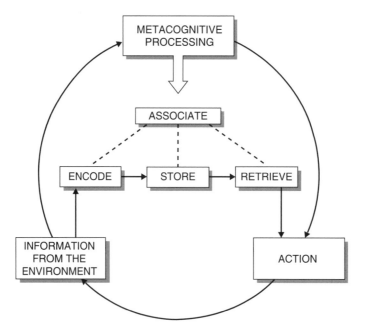

Figure 8.2 Simplified model of cognitive processing.

adapted to meet new, related demands. It is of little use if a stereotypical response occurs only in a certain context when specific cues are presented. Therapeutic interventions are often designed to emphasize cues, heighten feedback or give specific prompts and input at various points of task performance. Computers may be used to assist cognitive rehabilitation (McBain & Renton 1997).

At a higher level metacognition becomes important. This involves conscious organization and planning, and the ability to predict the results of one's actions.

Multicontext treatment approach

This uses very specific cognitive strategies to aid task performance. Treatment 'systematically changes task and environmental variables to enhance the person's ability to process, monitor and use information across new tasks and situations' (Toglia 1991 cited in Toglia 1998a). A similar approach to metacognitive training is described by Birnboim (1995).

Toglia presents a carefully structured approach in which there are five treatment components, each having associated actions to improve cognitive strategies and enable generalization of performance. The components are:

1. Specify a processing strategy for transfer of a behaviour from one situation to another.
2. Analyse tasks and establish criteria for transfer from one situation to another.
3. Practise application of the strategy in multiple environments and tasks.
4. Provide metacognitive training in self-monitoring and self-regulatory skills.
5. Take account of individual characteristics affecting motivation and active participation, and the degree of connection to previous learning.
(Adapted from Toglia 1998a)

Since the strategies used to promote learning and transfer of skills are complex and very specific the reader is advised to refer to the original texts and associated references.

Integrative micro/macro functional approach

This is a more generalized version of the cognitive approach (Duchek & Abreu 1997). The authors point out the importance of dealing with cognitive dysfunction from both 'bottom up' and 'top down' perspectives.

They state that, 'One assumption underlying this approach is that a relationship exists between the micro and macro levels of performance, and that this relationship is neither direct nor causal … the micro-macro approach is thus conceptualized as multidimensional and complex; it requires that therapists combine various methods from which a more effective and personalized assessment (and intervention) can develop'. A case example is provided to illustrate this.

The 'bottom up' approach focuses on cognitive performance components, whilst the 'top down' approach considers aspects such as personal meanings and motivations. Relevant assessments are listed.

Cognitive disability approach

This approach (Allen 1985 onward) is somewhat more evolved than the others and is described separately on page 107.

Outcome measures: There are numerous tests of memory and other aspects of cognition which provide specific measures. Standard functional ADL measures can also be used to detect improvements in performance.

Effectiveness: There is a considerable body of research literature in cognitive psychology. Because the use of these techniques within OT is relatively recent, literature is sparse. It should be possible to produce good supporting evidence by extracting relevant data from non-OT sources, but this has not yet been done systematically.

Advantages and disadvantages: The ability to learn and remember is an essential component of occupational performance. Application of cognitive theories and techniques, many of which have been extensively researched by psychologists and others, offers a promising avenue for specific intervention.

This approach is useful with cognitive deficits originating from physical or psychosocial causes.

Like all specialized AFRs, cognitive approaches require a very sound theoretical basis and expertise in the associated techniques, without which intervention is liable to be ineffective.

Because of the nature of the cognitive deficits affecting clients and the necessity for the therapist to define and control many aspects of intervention it is difficult for the therapist to use this approach in conjunction with a client-directed approach.

COGNITIVE BEHAVIOURAL AFR

This is a development from the behavioural AFR which, whilst still emphasizing the importance of the feedback from the results of behaviour on future actions, also takes account of the effects of thoughts and emotions on perceptions of the self as a competent and effective actor within the environment.

A number of cognitive approaches to the treatment of psychiatric illness or personality disorder have been developed. These approaches tend to emphasize the link between faulty ways of thinking and feeling or of perceiving the world, with various mental disorders, especially those associated with anxiety, depression and stress.

For example, Ellis introduced *rational emotive therapy*, summarized by the ABC theory: A is the Antecedent, a fact, event, behaviour or attitude which B influences the patient's Belief which C decides the Consequence. He also coined the expression 'musterbatory behaviour' to describe acts originating from irrational compulsive belief patterns.

Beck developed *cognitive therapy*, a less directive and interpretive style, based on helping the client to analyse the interactions of his thoughts, emotions and behaviours (Beck & Freeman 1990). Other workers look for 'life themes', persistent rules or attitudes which predominate in and direct the client's behaviour.

The individual's internal constructs of past, present, and particularly the future are of significance. The work of Bruner (a cognitive psychologist/educational theorist) has influenced the

models of some American OT theorists, especially his work on meaning as a component of human learning and behaviour (Bruner 1990).

Cognitive behavioural approaches are structured, and rely on methods which seek to change the content of thought, particularly anxious, depressive or obsessive thought patterns, thereby improving affect and behaviour.

Other approaches incorporate the theory of social modelling or techniques of behavioural rehearsal or role-play.

Primary assumptions

- Habitual, unnoticed, negative thoughts have a negative impact on behaviour.
- Negative thoughts make the individual feel bad about himself or some aspect of his life. Negative thoughts and feelings combine to lower expectations of personal control and efficacy.
- A cycle of dysfunction is set up (Fig. 8.3A) in which negative thoughts produce negative feelings which reduce expectance of success, reduce the effectiveness of performance and inhibit further attempts. A self-fulfilling prophesy of continued failure is established.
- This internal dynamic can be reversed if the client is enabled to use positive cognitive coping strategies. If negative thoughts can be challenged and replaced by positive ones action can be taken to solve problems. Performance therefore improves or is no longer viewed in negative terms. The individual gains positive feedback, begins to regain a sense of control and starts to feel good. This helps to inhibit negative thinking and feeds into a positive coping cycle (Fig. 8.3B).

Intervention strategies

These are aimed at breaking the negative cycle. In order to do this the therapist works with the client, either as an individual or, commonly, as a member of a group having similar problems, using the style of relationship described under Therapeutic alliance (p. 102). Techniques combine cognitive behavioural strategies and principles drawn from theories of adult education.

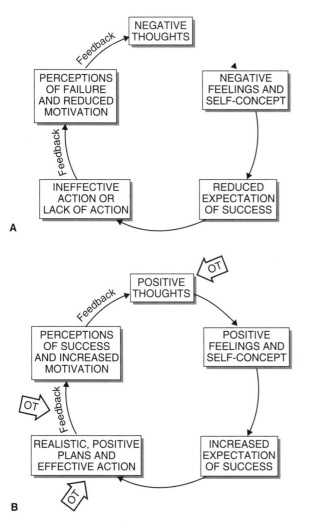

Figure 8.3 A Negative cognitive behavioural cycle; B positive cognitive behavioural cycle.

The therapist uses these practical problem-based techniques to help the individual to:

- Recognize negative emotions and the situations which provoke these
- Make the connection between negative emotions and habitual negative thoughts
- Identify negative thoughts, develop challenges to these and consciously evolve positive thoughts with which to replace them
- Explore values and attitudes which may contribute to the problem (such as unrealistically high expectations of self; adhering to rigid standards or routines;

denying oneself the opportunities for personal enjoyment)

- Recognize the ways in which negative thoughts and emotions inhibit adaptive action and limit performance
- Take control of daily life by setting realistic goals and working towards these in small, achievable steps
- Use problem-solving techniques to analyse problems and reduce them to manageable size in order to find solutions. These may include adaptations to task or environments or the acquisition of new skills and knowledge or conscious changes to mental attitudes, values and expectations
- Use techniques to manage stress
- Use techniques to improve communication with others
- Recognize personal achievements and reward self for them.

Active participation by the individual is essential. He may be asked to keep a diary or notebook, do assignments or practise specific techniques such as relaxation.

Other techniques such as anxiety management, behavioural rehearsal, coaching, scripting and role-play can be used.

This technique combines well with client-centred techniques of occupational analysis (Hagedorn 2000).

Evaluation of outcome: The individual reports and/or the therapist observes that goals have been achieved and a more adaptive cognitive cycle is developed. Overall increase in participation in a range of meaningful personal activities should be measured.

A number of psychometric tests such as measures of anxiety, depression or locus of control may be used as indicators.

Evidence of effectiveness: The psychological literature includes extensive research and description of the use of this technique.

Advantages and disadvantages: This is a very practical approach which focuses on present, meaningful issues in an individual's life and avoids any attempt at analysis or interpretation of unconscious material or intrapersonal dynamics. It is usually possible to promote change within a realistic timescale.

The techniques are not suitable for use with people with marked cognitive dysfunction or severe personality disorders.

ANALYTICAL AFR

The analytical AFR deals with the unconscious or subconscious basis of an individual's behaviour, his emotions and the personal meanings and symbolisms which he may attribute to people, events or objects. This hidden material may be uncovered by a variety of techniques. This AFR can be used with an individual in a dyadic relationship with the therapist or with individuals loosely organized in a group.

The classic form of psychoanalysis is that originated by Freud at the beginning of the 20th century. He created the terms which have passed into the language of analysis – e.g. unconscious, preconscious, id, ego, super-ego, libido – and proposed that the gratification of drives, especially sexuality, was the basis of human behaviour. The development of the individual during infancy and childhood follows a series of stages. Fixation in or regression to one of these early stages limits the development of an integrated personality.

Other schools of psychoanalysis have developed subsequently, extending or deviating from Freud's original explanations of the basis of human personality. A significant theory considers 'object relations' – the perceptions of and relationships with people or desired objects, particularly as a baby – to have a fundamental influence on subsequent relationships and behaviour.

Psychoanalysts view the individual as being motivated by unconscious drives and emotions which direct behaviour and are not subject to voluntary control. Some of these unconscious forces are innate, others arise through the interpretation of past experiences, usually as a very young child. The individual can by a long process of analysis, during which the relationship with the analyst is a significant part of therapy, come to a better (but never complete)

understanding of the reasons for his feelings and behaviour and this may help him to live a more satisfying and less anxious life. The analytical approach, therefore, takes a primarily retrospective view of human actions, understanding of the past bringing comprehension of the present and removing anxieties concerning the future.

Since Freud, many theorists have developed their own ideas following one or other of the above styles, or attempted a synthesis. The role of the analyst varies from the neutral to the directive and from the reflective to the actively interpretive or interactive. There are far too many notable names to mention them all, but some people who have produced innovatory and influential theories between the First and Second World Wars include:

- Freud (stages of sexuality; gratification of drives)
- Adler (will to power)
- Jung (dreams and symbols; archetypes and the collective unconscious)
- Klein (object relations; infantile experiences)
- Sullivan (object relations; juvenile anxiety)
- Winnicott (child/mother relationship)
- Guntrip (repressed ego).

Later theorists are even more numerous and the student is advised to read texts selectively to avoid becoming confused by elaborate and contradictory concepts.

Primary assumptions: This summary deals with broad principles shared by the main schools of analysis as interpreted in the context of OT. In analytical practice there are marked differences between theorists which are reflected in the use of language and techniques.

- Behaviour is governed by unconscious, irrational processes, linked to the gratification of basic drives.
- Early life, during which a person develops through psychosexual stages, or stages in the development of relationships with persons and objects, has a lasting effect on personality.
- Conflicts, anxiety, guilt, depression or problems with relationships in later life are symptoms of unresolved unconscious

conflicts originating in repressed memories of infancy and childhood.

- Subconscious material may surface in the form of dreams and symbols which may affect perceptions of reality.
- It is possible through a lengthy process of analysis to uncover the origins of symptoms, to bring material out of the unconscious, to gain insight, and thereby to resolve conflicts, anxieties and unsatisfactory relationships (Fig. 8.4).

Terminology: Patient/client; analysand; therapist; analyst; therapy; analysis (and the language of the particular theorist, e.g. Freud: ego, superego, libido, transference, countertransference, projection, repression, unconscious, preconscious).

Patient/therapist relationship: It is anticipated that a complex relationship occurs during an extended process of analysis which involves mechanisms such as projection, transference and countertransference. Although the occupational therapist is not functioning as an analyst, such relationships may develop, and the therapist must be aware of his own mechanisms of defence or transference. The patient may develop some dependency on the therapist.

Advantages and disadvantages: Focuses on emotions and relationships; releases unconscious material and makes it accessible. Recognizes an irrational basis for behaviour.

Since the process is highly subjective it can be hard to define goals or the problem. The process is usually slow; results may not be apparent until months or even years after therapeutic interventions or experiences. The patient may become dependent on the therapist. Traditional Freudian thinking fosters a submissive female stereotype judged by the standards of current Western culture (neo-Freudians have modified accordingly). For the occupational therapist, use of dynamic techniques requires expertise: overinterpretation or misinterpretation by the therapist could be misleading or damaging. Releasing unconscious material without dealing with it appropriately may produce violent emotional reactions and behaviours. Techniques may be stressful for the therapist if he uncovers personal material or emotions.

Projective techniques approach

When using this approach the occupational therapist typically uses creative and projective techniques such as art, sculpture, drama or mime, working with people as individuals or as a collection of individuals within a group. The person's reactions to and interpretation of his creative endeavours help to uncover hidden symbolisms or emotions. Discussion of these provides insight into underlying psychological mechanisms such as repression, denial, guilt, conflict or projection. This works best with intelligent, articulate patients who have a degree of insight.

Material which is brought to the surface has to be dealt with – worked through – so that the patient can acknowledge and cope with it. Repressed material is dangerous from the client's point of view – that is why it was repressed in the first place. It triggers uncomfortable emotions such as guilt, anxiety, sexual desires or anger, and exploration of all this can only be done, if at all, in a safe environment. This sense of trust and safety has to be created by the therapist.

Although clients may work within a group, they usually do so as individuals, not as group members. Analytical theories are concerned with the reasons for an individual's reactions to her own feelings or to other individuals or objects, not with his reactions to people in general or groups as a whole.

The degree to which an occupational therapist may interpret the use of images and symbols by the client and the manner in which the therapist facilitates self-discovery depends on the theory within which he is working, and the techniques with which he is familiar. Sometimes it is the client's interpretations which are used, sometimes it may be those of the therapist, but interpretations are suggested, not imposed.

Psychoanalytical approaches

The occupational therapist is not, and should not try to be, a psychoanalyst or psychotherapist.

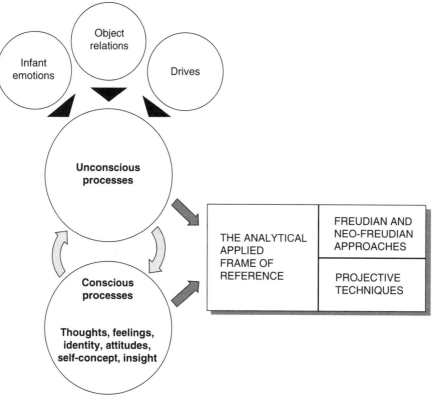

Figure 8.4 Analytical applied frame of reference.

Because of the highly potent nature of unconscious material all psychoanalytical techniques should be used with discretion, following suitable training, and the practitioner must have access to adequate personal supervision. (The supervisor must be a person suitably qualified both to oversee the therapist's treatment of patients and also to deal with the dynamics of the therapist's own needs, dilemmas and personal growth.) The material which a patient produces needs to be dealt with by a properly qualified analyst.

The analytical approach was first developed by Fidler in the USA; she was interested in the potential of activities for releasing reactions and emotions and acting as a vehicle for communication between therapist and client – hence her approach is sometimes called 'the communication approach'. The most frequently described approaches are: psychodynamic (analytical)

approach (Levy 1993); object relations approach (Mosey 1986).

GROUP WORK AFR

The group work AFR is based on theories concerning the dynamics of group interactions and processes and their effects on the behaviour and reactions of group members (Fig. 8.5). In this AFR the group is the important entity, and all individual experiences are explored through the medium of the group. It is possible to have groups which are analytically based, but also to use other approaches, such as cognitive or humanistic, within a group setting. In OT the group may focus on some activity as a means of facilitating the group process.

In psychiatric settings there are two aspects to this AFR which may or may not overlap: firstly, a concern with the individual's skills

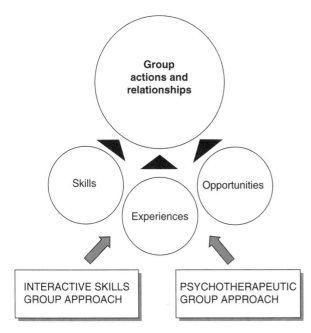

Figure 8.5 Group work applied frame of reference.

of interpersonal communication (interactive approach/activities group approach); and, secondly, a concern with the ability of an individual to function as a member of a group, and the power of the group to function as a therapeutic entity (psychotherapeutic group approach).

Interactive skills approach

Primary assumptions: The skills of interacting with other people can only be acquired experientially.

Certain basic interactive skills must be acquired before an individual can form relationships or function competently as a member of a group.

Shared involvement in group activities and projects, creative, social or recreational, promotes skill development and social learning.

This form of group is structured to promote the development and use of interpersonal and social skills. The therapist will assess deficits in verbal and non-verbal communication, personal appearance and cultural appropriateness and will design situations and exercises which will promote the ability of the client to initiate and

sustain appropriate and effective interactions with other individuals, to recognize and express her own needs, and to take account of the needs of others.

This is based on cognitive and experiential methods, not behavioural ones, although the approach may also include skills training, particularly social interactive skills, communicative skills and skills in assertion. This may begin dyadically with individuals who are unable to cope with being in a group, but such techniques are most often used in a group setting where members can interact and experiment.

Mosey (1986) describes the use of activity groups in detail and lists a number of types: evaluative, task orientated, developmental and thematic. She also describes formats for developmental groups, each one involving the patient in a higher level of communication and cooperation: parallel, egocentric-cooperative, project, cooperative, mature.

The choice of activity and the arrangement of the environment in which the group takes place are crucial in promoting the right level of interaction.

Examples of techniques
- Social activities
- Social games, quizzes, etc.
- Group projects
- Creative activities
- Role-play
- Social/communication skills training.

Outcome measures: Individual group members are likely to have personal goals related to improvements in social skills. Assessments may measure improvements specifically or in more general functional terms.

Effectiveness: Group settings have long been accepted as an effective milieu for social learning. Evidence that a particular structure for the group or involvement in one activity rather than another is more or less effective may be harder to come by.

Advantages and disadvantages: Activities groups are a practical way to involve clients in situations which promote acquisition of social skills. Social learning requires a structured environment and careful facilitation; it will not necessarily take place when clients are simply 'having a good time' in a recreational setting. Organization of effective activity groups is time consuming.

Psychotherapeutic group approach

Primary assumptions
- Interaction with other people in structured therapeutic groups provides a means of achieving personal growth and insight and developing interactive skills.
- The group process is in itself a dynamic and potent therapeutic medium.
- Personal growth is a painful process which requires a secure and supportive group environment.
- Group work can facilitate communication and cohesion between group members and provides a means of dealing with conflicts.

Terminology: Client; therapist; co-therapist; group leader; facilitator; closed group; open group; group process; group dynamic; activity group.

Group therapy is based on theories of group dynamics and may borrow or adapt techniques derived from psychotherapeutic practice. There is a wide spectrum of types of groups, from relatively unstructured, open groups to closed psychotherapy groups which operate over an extended period with a fixed number of participants, and which may or may not involve task-related activity.

It is typical of this form of group work that the product of group activity, whilst giving the group a focus and a potential sense of achievement, is subordinate to the group process, which provides the insights and learning experiences for group members and gives the therapist opportunities to explore both individual issues and group dynamics.

There may be a degree of interpretation and analysis of the dynamics of interactions, or the results of participation in activities, but often the main purpose of the group is to provide opportunities for clients to participate in order to explore their personal reactions and problems by means of interactions and shared group processes or to improve their abilities to communicate their own needs and to be sensitive to those of others.

The role of the therapist in facilitating this process, and the style of leadership used, are crucial. A group takes time to form, to reach a point where members function as a group and not as individuals, and even longer to reach a point where it really performs. Therapeutic groups are essentially artificial creations and can be difficult to manage – there is a great deal of scope for conflict; the group may disintegrate, split into cliques or get sidelined away from important issues. A therapist needs to be very experienced and knowledgeable about group theory and group techniques to manage conflicts constructively and get the best out of a group. A good group is cohesive, mutually supportive, goal orientated and productive. When a group really does gel the results can be exciting.

Techniques
- Role-play
- Gaming
- Projective techniques
- Psychodrama
- Assertion training
- Anxiety management
- Stress management
- Communication skills training
- Social skills training.

Outcome measures: It is likely to be difficult to express outcome measures in a quantitative form. Predetermined personal goals or objectives for participants should be met. In some settings the group itself will determine whether the outcome is successful in whichever way they choose to define this.

Effectiveness: Evidence is more likely to be found within psychotherapy literature than in OT.

Advantages and disadvantages: When well led or facilitated, group work can produce good results. Working with people in groups is an effective use of resources. The group process is experiential and highly relevant to the client;

although beneficial results may be slow to appear they tend to be long-lasting.

A group needs to meet several times to be effective. A psychotherapeutic group may need to continue for several months and results may not appear until long after the group is ended. Group management – whichever style of leadership or facilitation is employed – is highly skilled. Group work is stressful for the therapist, who must have additional training and access to supervision.

CLIENT-CENTRED AFR

Humanistic psychology needs to be distinguished from 'humanism' which is a philosophy concerned with the nature of humanity, personal consciousness and individual being. Humanism influenced the development of humanistic psychology and humanistic educational theory. Humanism takes a strongly atheistic stand-point; however, humanistic psychology does not preclude religious belief.

Humanistic psychology is described as phenomenological because it is concerned with subjective individual experience, the personal 'world view' that each individual develops as a result of his unique life, feelings and perceptions.

Influential theorists are Maslow (self-actualization), Frankl (personal meaning), Kelly (personal construct) and Rogers (person-centred counselling and person-centred learning).

These theorists emphasize the essentially positive nature of every individual, who should be valued and will respond accordingly. The individual has the potential to control her life and to choose what she wishes to become. She can only change and progress if she wills to do so; change can only take place if it is an active process which is meaningful to the individual. Positive change can occur throughout life. Living should be a celebratory, joyful experience.

Important concepts in the humanistic view of personal relationships are the need for authenticity (being one's true self), honesty and non-judgemental regard and respect for others. These theories have become very influential in psychotherapy, teaching, social work and OT, and linked with some developmental and cognitive theories. There are many natural resonances between person-centred theories and the fundamental philosophy of OT as expressed by its American founders (long before humanistic psychology had been developed).

Carl Rogers has been very significant in the move from teacher/therapist-centred, directive approaches to student/client-centred ones. He felt that therapists should act as counsellors or facilitators, providing resources and enabling people to learn and change. He saw learning as a life-long search for individual meaning, fulfilment, growth and self-knowledge. His ideas were based on personal experience as a teacher and counsellor, backed up by the anecdotal accounts of others.

Key features of Rogerian counselling or psychotherapy are that it is person centred, uses a non-directive style, avoids interpretation, reflects back to the individual her ideas, perceptions and beliefs and provides encouragement to search for personal meaning and self-actualization. Practitioners believe that it is theoretically possible, by means of counselling, for an individual to achieve a large degree of self-knowledge and control over her own life.

The humanistic perspective has been criticized for promoting unrealistic starry-eyed optimism and, whilst the ideals are given lip-service by many, they are frequently not put into practice, not least because many of the systems within which health care is delivered make it difficult to allow the amount of time and the degree of freedom of choice for the client which is required. In reality, the opportunity for the individual to control, direct and shape her own life may be minimal and, whilst choice may be beneficial, some clients are overwhelmed by being presented with too much of it.

The amount of expertise and training required to use humanistic techniques such as client-centred counselling is also frequently underestimated. Whilst basic counselling skills can be acquired quite readily by most therapists, it should be recognized that clients requiring long-term or indepth counselling should be referred to a suitably qualified counsellor or psychotherapist.

A number of holistic, humanistic psychotherapies have evolved, frequently combining elements of cognitive or developmental theories with humanism and psychotherapy, including:

- Gestalt therapy (Perls)
- Rational emotive therapy (Ellis)
- Personal construct (repertory grid) (Kelly; Bannister & Fransella)
- Transactional analysis (Berne)
- Psychosynthesis (Assagioli)
- Person-centred counselling (Maslow; Rogers)
- Encounter groups (Rogers)
- Co-counselling (Jackins)
- Theme-centred group work (Cohn).

In the context of OT, the humanistic AFR has produced distinct approaches, including: the client-directed approach (incorporating various person-centred counselling techniques) and the student-centred approach (based largely on Rogerian principles of education).

Client-centred approaches

What is a client?

A client, in the traditional definition, is a person who seeks the services of a professional person. By implication a client has a reason to seek these services, and a desire to be active in resolving some situation in his life with which the knowlege or skills of the professional person may help. There is, therefore, a mutual expectation and contract, formal or informal, between the client and the professional person. The client expects good advice and competent professional services. The provider expects to gain an understanding of the problem and to be able to do something about it. The relationship between client and professional has a distinct purpose and precise boundaries.

In health care 'client' has been used as an opposite designation to 'patient'. Patients are passive, dependent and in a subordinate role in relation to the professional person. The patient says, 'I'm here, do what you can to make me better; I'll do whatever you say'. The client, in contrast, says, 'What I want is this … tell me what you can offer me, let us discuss this; I may or may not decide to do as you suggest.'

It is worth noting, however, that in the traditional view of the relationship between a client and a professional person, the professional is usually in a position of giving some kind of expert advice. In the client-centred AFR this may not necessarily be the case.

'Client-centred' has become a somewhat over-used phrase in recent years, and along with words associated with it, is subject to a range of interpretations. It is a mistake to consider this AFR as homogenous, since different approaches are used within it.

A significant distinction between this AFR and others is that it is focused on the style of relationship between client and therapist, or between teacher and student, rather than on explanations of physical or psychosocial dysfunction.

Fundamentally this AFR is based on humanistic ideals and principles.

Primary assumptions

- The personal experience and consciousness of the individual is of paramount importance; since no one else can experience it, no one should attempt to influence another's choices or interpretations of reality.
- The individual must be considered as a whole in the context of his physical and social environment.
- An individual has the right to personal choice (and all other human rights).
- The goal of the individual is to be autonomous, authentic and self-actualizing (functioning as a free, self-directing, honest person whose life brings self-satisfaction and contains personal meaning).
- The individual is capable of controlling events in her life and should direct her own education or therapy as far as possible.
- An individual is innately capable of positive development.

The client-centred AFR has given rise to four related approaches:

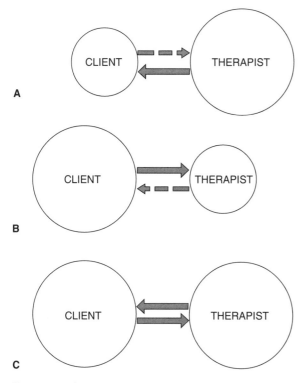

Figure 8.6 Client-centred approaches: **A** person-centred ethical practice; **B** client-directed approach; **C** therapeutic alliance (and student-centred approach).

1. The person-centred ethical practice approach
2. The client-directed approach
3. The therapeutic alliance approach
4. The student-centred educational approach.

These may be conceptualized as indicating different weighting of the roles of client and therapist (Fig. 8.6).

Person-centred ethical practice approach

In some areas of therapeutic practice the therapist works with potentially vulnerable people whose ability to take personal decisions or to contribute in any substantial or meaningful way to the organization of their daily lives is very limited. Examples might include people with severe learning difficulties, people with advanced dementia and those with serious brain injury.

The person-centred ethical practice approach, whilst recognizing that these clients have many limitations, demands that the therapist should regard each individual as unique and valuable. The individual must have his human rights protected and respected. He must be treated with personal respect and dignity at all times. There should be a positive expectation that the client will be involved in decisions about his life and given opportunities and choices, just as much as if he were fully able.

This ethically based approach was evolved during the early 1980s to counteract bad practice in which persons dependent on care or confined within an institution were deprived of basic rights, not through malign intention but because of institutionalized attitudes, depersonalizing authoritarian regimes and associated use of patronizing language. Substantial efforts were made at that time to normalize living conditions, and improve the quality of life for residents in care, redesigning the environment to remove all the institutional trappings which might reinforce negative attitudes. This approach continued and developed as the move towards community care progressed. It is associated with social role valorization and gentle teaching (Webber 1995).

These ideals are now widely accepted and have become standard practice in most care settings. However, difficult ethical problems and dilemmas still arise, and the approach has to be supported by good management, with appropriate policies and safeguards against abuse.

The therapist may sometimes need to act as an advocate for the client, communicating his needs and wishes to others and putting over the client's point of view on his behalf.

Effectiveness: This approach changes attitudes, and therefore affects the behaviour of carers and other professionals in ways which improve the quality of care. Failure to provide high standards of person-centred, ethically based care would now be regarded as questionable.

Client-directed approach

This approach is derived from theories and techniques developed for non-directive, person-centred counselling and psychotherapy.

In this approach the client is in control. The client sets the parameters, decides on goals, works out personal priorities, and then plans action to achieve these. Through the growing experience of control and mastery, the client is enabled to change and develop in ways which are meaningful to him.

The therapist is there to empower and enable the client to steer this process. She may offer opportunities for discussion, enabling the client to explore personal needs, thoughts and feelings and to construct goals. Various person-centred counselling techniques may be used to facilitate this process. Once goals have been set, the therapist tries to enable action by the client, providing support, encouragement and resources which the client identifies as necessary.

Whilst the therapist may help the client to explore or question aspects of his life she does not impose her own judgements (even when the client, in the therapist's personal view, has 'got it wrong'). Only by starting from the point where the client is, and by dealing with things as he sees them, can one help him to move onward. In order to 'be with' the client the therapist must submerge her own sense of self within an empathic understanding of what it means to be the other person.

Outcome measures: The outcome is evaluated by the client, although the therapist may assist by providing outcome measures which the client can use to do this (e.g. the Canadian Occupational Performance Measure).

Effectiveness: From the perspective of service delivery, this is not an easy approach. The techniques can be time-consuming and results may be hard to evaluate. Whilst it is recognized that the quality of the therapeutic relationship influences outcomes evidence of superior effectiveness of this style of interaction is inconclusive; it is intrinsically hard to evaluate objectively.

Advantages and disadvantages: A person who has found a way to do the things which are important to him, in the way he wants to do them, and has 'taken charge' is likely to regard the outcome positively, and to build adaptively on these changes.

The development of the client's sense of personal identity, self-efficacy and self-actualization is, however, a highly demanding process. It depends on the client's ability to learn, adapt and be in contact with reality. Where these abilities are reduced, progress is likely to be very slow.

The method depends heavily on the quality of the therapeutic relationship. It may take a long time for the client to reach the point where goal planning, prioritizing and subsequent action become possible. The client may have come to the therapist precisely because he finds these things very difficult. There is a danger that the process may slide into rather fuzzy, 'all talk, no do' mode.

It is difficult to reconcile a client-directed approach with the value systems and practical constraints of medical-model clinical settings. The lack of direction from the therapist may make some clients (and, indeed, some therapists) feel unsure rather than empowered. Since the client is in control, failure to make progress may conveniently be attributed to a failure of the client rather than to a failure of the therapist to facilitate the relationship and develop the process.

The client-directed approach is not occupationally based and this element has to be introduced by the therapist, otherwise the OT focus can easily become blurred or lost.

Therapeutic alliance

In this approach the client and therapist come together in search of a way to resolve problems or move the situation forward. The relationship is based on mutual respect, valuing each other's input, and a shared desire to achieve an outcome. This is sometimes described as a partnership. This style of relationship is increasingly in use in health care by a wide range of professions including doctors, especially in settings where a social model of service provision is in use.

In the context of OT the word 'partnership' refers to mutual engagement in a shared enterprise, that of helping the client to identify and achieve his occupational goals. There is an implication of equality, but this has to be set in context.

Therapist and client are equal in the way that all humans are equal, and from this perspective the partnership must strive for equilibrium within the therapeutic relationship (see Fig. 8.6C). The two partners are not necessarily equal in other respects. Each may contribute more or less of certain aspects of the therapeutic alliance, but both participants have something to contribute.

The client is the expert on his own situation. He knows what has happened to him, what he has experienced, and what he seeks. He has knowledge and skills, but may also recognize that he needs more to meet the challenges of his situation. He sees the therapist as a resource who may have something to contribute.

The therapist brings special knowledge and skills, and access to information or resources. It is important for the therapist to begin by making a clear, concise explanation of what services she can (and cannot) provide, 'setting out her stall' so that the client can see what is on offer and make an informed choice. She can enable and empower the client in his search. She will both encourage him to act and, if mutually agreed, take some action for him.

The therapist may challenge or question the client's views, and may give advice or suggest alternatives, respecting the client's ultimate right to disagree or to refuse to accept what she offers. The client may, equally, challenge the therapist; being a professional does not imply any automatic right to superior judgement or continual infallibility. The therapist must be prepared to acknowledge when she does not have an answer.

After a period of mutual exploration of the problem which has caused the client to seek the services of the therapist, goals are negotiated and agreed, solutions explored and an action plan decided on. Action may be taken by the client or the therapist or both.

This type of approach was proposed by Schon (1983) as a contract between the reflective practitioner and her client, as distinct from the traditional style of contract between expert and patient in which the authority resides firmly with the professional.

Outcome measures: Outcomes are evaluated by both partners using a pre-arranged format appropriate to the situation.

A wide range of outcome measures can be used within this approach, provided that the client participates actively in the process and shares with the therapist the task of attempting to understand and use the results.

Effectiveness: Evidence of whether this approach works more or less effectively than others remains sketchy.

Advantages and disadvantages: This is a flexible and pragmatic version of the client-centred AFR which is compatible with problem-based approaches. It can be used within rehabilitation settings where the social model is in use, and works well in community settings.

In more traditional clinical settings there is a danger that this compromise approach may become a watered-down version of the client-centred AFR, simply being used as window-dressing for a more user-friendly version of the traditional approach without really adopting the underlying person-centred attitudes and values.

The notion of partnership has been criticized as invalid by McColl et al (1997), on the basis that the therapeutic partnership is not a true mutual sharing of gains or liabilities, since the risk remains with the client.

On the other hand, it might equally be argued that, whilst both parties can celebrate gains, both parties share equally in responsibility for failure.

Student-centred educational approach

As an educational approach this has been in wide use since the mid-1980s especially with adult learners.

There is a range of styles of relationship between teacher and student, from very non-directive educational approaches in which the teacher plays a relatively passive and responsive role to partnership approaches which operate on the same principles as the therapeutic alliance.

In student-centred learning it is usual for the student to set personal learning objectives, plan a means of achieving these, and evaluate how far they have been achieved.

The teacher acts as a sounding board enabling the student to test ideas, validate concepts and identify the need for additional learning.

Advantages and disadvantages are similar to those described for the other approaches, but transferred to an educational context.

9

Applied frames of reference developed by named practitioners

The AFRs so far described, although widely used by occupational therapists, have been evolved as a kind of corporate endeavour by the profession as a whole. There is usually no named author.

There have been some AFRs, however, which have been presented or originated by an individual therapist. These differ from the occupational performance models described in the final section in that they take a more narrowly focused view, considering just one aspect or theory or the needs of a client group.

Examples of AFR for use with children and with adults with developmental disorders are given in Box 9.1 but will not be described further.

Two theorists have been influential in work with adults in mental health settings. These are Anne Cronin Mosey, who was one of the first therapists to present a set of frames of reference for use in the context of psychosocial dysfunction, and Claudia Allen whose cognitive disabilities frame of reference was originated for use in

---

Box 9.1 Frames of reference for use with children or adults with developmental disorders

AFR	Original author and date
Sensory Integration	Ayres (1973) (see Kielhofner 1992; Miller & Walker 1993; Baloueff 1998)
Developmental: Facilitating growth and development	Llorens (1970; 1976) (see Miller & Walker 1993)
Spatiotemporal adaptation	Gilfoyle, Grady (1983) (see Kielhofner 1992)

long-term psychiatry but has found application in other areas.

THREE FRAMES OF REFERENCE FOR PSYCHOSOCIAL DYSFUNCTION (MOSEY)

All three frames of reference deal with the use of activities as vehicles for skill or role development.

The *analytical frame of reference* is described as being appropriate when dealing with a client whose life situation involves difficulties with 'universal issues'. These are listed as: reality, trust, intimacy, adequacy, dependence/independence, sexuality and aggression. Her interpretation of the analytical approach is eclectic but appears to be based more on object relations theories than Freudian ones.

The *acquisitional frame of reference* has a cognitive/behavioural base, and deals mainly with the acquisition of interpersonal skills and roles.

In *recapitulation of ontogenesis* Mosey uses a developmental/humanist frame of reference but links this with elements of cognitive and social learning theory. She identifies six (originally seven; drive-object skill was removed from later lists) *adaptive skills*. These skills are acquired sequentially and are universal. They include:

- Perceptual motor skill. The ability to receive, select, combine and coordinate vestibular, proprioceptive and tactile information for functional use
- Cognitive skill. The ability to perceive, represent and organize sensory information for the purpose of thinking and problem solving
- Dyadic interaction skill. The ability to participate in a variety of dyadic relationships
- Group interaction skill. The ability to engage in a variety of primary groups
- Self-identity skill. The ability to perceive the self as a relatively autonomous, holistic and acceptable person who has permanence and continuity over time
- Sexual identity skill. The ability to perceive one's sexual nature as good and to participate

in a relatively long-term sexual relationship that is oriented to the mutual satisfaction of sexual needs (Mosey 1986). Note: this list is taken from her most recent publication, and differs in some small but significant aspects from her previous definitions.

These adaptive skills are composed of *adaptive subskills* which in turn are composed of *skill components*. Perhaps the most interesting and potentially useful part of the model is the analysis of each of the six skills as a developmental sequence, linked to chronological developmental stages in which each skill evolves in complexity and adaptive potential. An assessment of the level of function therefore enables one to determine a developmental age or level for the individual in each skill. This enables activities and interactions to be selected at the correct level so that early skills can be learnt or regained before later ones and the correct developmental sequence is retained. This is similar to the approach of Allen (1985), who proposes a cognitive/developmental system using very well structured activities aimed at identified levels.

Assessments and interventions are related to each of these areas, depending on the type of dysfunction, and a range of standardized tests is proposed.

In common with Reed and Kielhofner, Mosey quotes Reilly (see Miller & Walker 1993) and emphasizes the use of activity, both for individuals and in structured groups. Experiential learning through activity, interactions and group work is seen as the means of producing adaptive responses or improving skills.

Like Reed, she is concerned with 'wellness' rather than 'illness' and suggests a list of health needs which a therapist should be aware of and should attempt to meet through OT programmes. Because her base is in psychiatric practice, the purpose of this list seems largely to be to foster anti-institutionalized relationships and programmes.

This list has similarities with Maslow's hierarchy of needs, and includes:

- Psychophysical needs (physiological, environmental)

- Temporal balance and regularity (varied pattern of occupations and timing)
- Safety (physical and emotional)
- Love and acceptance (client/therapist relationship)
- Group association (sharing)
- Mastery (successful participation in activity)
- Esteem (a valued, rewarding role)
- Sexual needs (recognizing needs; enabling needs to be met)
- Pleasure (client's individual definition)
- Self-actualization (meaningful activities and relationships).

Mosey presents a detailed and densely argued account of OT which cannot be encapsulated in a few pages. Her ideas are pragmatic and those who find them interesting are recommended to try and obtain her book. (Mosey does not give a visual representation of her ideas, and it would be presumptuous to invent one.)

Advantages and disadvantages: Mosey offers a flexible and non-dogmatic approach widely applicable in psychosocial dysfunction. It is activity based. It recognizes that progress cannot be achieved if the individual has not reached the required developmental level. The therapist identifies the level and assists correct choice of activity in the correct sequence. This is particularly useful for individuals functioning at a lower developmental level.

The strongly psychosocial emphasis leads to restricted applicability in physical settings.

THE COGNITIVE DISABILITY AFR (ALLEN)

This AFR has been developed over the past 20 years in the USA by Claudia Allen, originally as an alternative approach for the treatment of chronic psychiatric disorders, especially those resulting in impairments to the individual's ability to cope with basic daily tasks.

Allen realized that the rehabilitation process, with its implied expectation of recovery, and the traditional focus on 'stretching abilities' as a means of achieving improvement, did not produce the expected results in patients with chronic disorders in which cognitive function was diminished or liable to decline.

Drawing on theories from cognitive, developmental and biological perspectives in psychology, this perception led her to challenge the applicability of the concepts on which traditional therapy was based. Her conclusions were considered radical when she first proposed them and are still viewed by some as controversial.

She developed the concept of cognitive disability: 'a restriction in voluntary motor action originating in the physical or chemical structures of the brain and producing observable limitations in routine task behaviour' (Allen 1985).

She hypothesized that a cognitive disability was due to actual brain damage, be it chemical (temporary or permanent) or anatomical. This damage reduced normal function. Six levels related to cognitive function could be observed and described (Box 9.2).

Allen uses information-processing models of cognition, and describes the following factors as contributing to task performance: attention to sensory cues; motor actions; conscious awareness; purpose; experience; process; time.

The crucial, and at the time controversial, part of her theory was the view that an individual could only function within the limits of his/her cognitive level and could not be expected to function above this level unless some fundamental change occurred as a result of medication or the remission of illness. She created task-related tests by means of which the level of cognitive function could be assessed.

Allen states her rationale quite boldly: 'Therapists might assume that a description of six levels will direct our services towards increasing the cognitive level. Implicit in the assumption is a question: can occupational therapy change the cognitive level? The answer is no, at least for the present' (Allen 1985).

She goes on to suggest that it is pointless to bewilder and frustrate individuals with cognitive disabilities by presenting them with challenging tasks or situations to which they are unable to respond. Instead, she proposes that tasks, tools and environment need to be structured very precisely to compensate for deficits and produce optimum performance at each level.

Since this initial presentation of her theories, Allen has refined and evolved them, and they have been applied in fields other than psychiatry, e.g. the treatment of head injuries, strokes, learning disabilities, dementia and other disorders where cognitive disability is a feature.

Task analysis and environmental analysis

At each level different forms of tasks, presentation of information, tools and materials, and arrangement of environmental cues are required. These are described in detail and are of interest beyond the confines of the AFR, providing a clear example of the occupational therapist's approach to the therapeutic application and adaptation of activities.

Perhaps because the approach was generated in the context of long-stay psychiatry, Allen has developed the use of simple craft projects typically employed in large institutions, both as illustrations of the necessary adaptations for each level, and also as a means of assessment.

Whilst some have welcomed this specific use of traditional crafts, therapists who are less drawn to the making of mosaic trivets and leather thonging have found this restricting; however, the general approach can readily be adapted for use with simple daily living tasks such as cooking.

Assessments

The Allen Cognitive Level (ACL) test uses performance at leather lacing (thonging) as a test of cognitive ability.

This task is too complex for some patients and the lower cognitive level test, which asks the patient to imitate the action of clapping, was designed for patients at levels 1, 2 or 3.

The routine task inventory (RTI) is a daily living checklist rated by interview and/or observation, with four subscales dealing with areas of work, communication, physical activity and communication.

These assessments are marketed in the UK together with a manual and use does not require special training.

Approach

The cognitive disabilities AFR mainly uses a compensatory approach, seeking to maximize residual function through task adaptation and environmental adaptation. The emphasis is on adapting the task and the circumstances of performance to match the abilities of the individual, rather than expecting the individual to change or adapt.

Allen locates the points at which change can be made in the life of an individual (structure; process; environment) and shows how the adaptive models, which expect the patient to make changes to meet new demands, are inappropriate for people who are unable to cope with new learning, and for whom a 'magical cure' is unlikely.

Outcome measures: Allen and her colleagues have developed a set of task-based assessments which provide indications of the cognitive level at which the client is functioning. Standard functional assessments may also be used, provided that the tasks are pitched at the appropriate cognitive level. Improvements in performance of these tasks might indicate improvement in cognition, but should also indicate that adaptations to tasks and environments have successfully enabled the client to perform to his or her maximum potential.

Effectiveness: Research into the effectiveness of this approach is being conducted. A search of current literature should produce some evidence.

Advantages and disadvantages: Allen recognizes the reality that some people cannot change adaptively, have limited abilities and require special help to maximize their residual skills. She proposes a simple set of diagnostic assessments. The concepts are coherent and well explained. The approach removes the sense of professional frustration resulting from failure to achieve 'improvement'.

It is possible that, in institutional settings, the reductive nature of the approach may result in

---

Box 9.2   Six cognitive levels

Level 1: Reflexive (automatic actions) The individual seems unaware of external environment or stimuli. Only simple, single, automated, gross patterns of movement are initiated. No constructive tasks can be attempted; one word instructions may trigger an automatic response. Actions are not imitated if demonstrated.

Level 2: Movement (postural actions) The individual attends to her own movement, or that of others, or of objects. Movement follows simple gross motor patterns, e.g. pacing, rocking, with no purpose except seeking comfort. Some actions may be imitated, but little or no purposeful task performance is achieved.

Level 3: Repetitive actions (manual actions) Objects are the centre of attention, and are repetitively explored or manipulated, but with little purpose. Objects are recognized as separate from self, but the patient is unaware of others and is generally disorientated. Very simple repetitive actions may be attempted under close instruction and supervision but attention span is very short.

Level 4: End product (goal directed actions) The individual is able to pay attention to the tangible elements of her environment as long as these are within view and reach. A thing out of sight 'disappears' and will not be looked for. A very familiar repetitive task can be completed, or a simple pattern or demonstration followed slowly, one step at a time, with verbal cues. Task completion brings satisfaction. Judgement is poor and problem solving virtually non-existent.

Level 5: Variations (exploratory actions) Allen says that a percentage of the 'normal' population functions at this level. The individual is able to initiate actions to achieve personal goals, and can adjust actions as the task progresses to some extent, e.g. finding missing item but has trouble planning ahead, anticipating or solving problems except by trial and error. Personal needs come first, and the person does not usually think before she acts, or pause to consider the consequences.

Level 6: Tangible thought (planned actions) The individual is capable of symbolic thought, uses reasoning and problem solving and is capable of showing initiative and creativity. Complex activities and chains of activities can be completed. Level 6 is associated with a higher educational and occupational background.

---

a patient becoming labelled, e.g. as a 'level 3'; this may negatively affect staff perceptions and result in self-fulfilling prophecies of low performance, and failure to recognize change due to chemotherapy or remission of illness (certainly not what the author intended). The approach has a narrow theoretical base and discounts other explanations for dysfunction, e.g. motivational ones. The dogmatic statement that OT cannot improve cognition requires further research.

Processes of change

10

Processes of change

DEVELOPMENT, ADAPTATION, REHABILITATION AND EDUCATION

From the moment an individual is born he becomes subject to processes of change. Changes occur as part of normal growth, maturation and ageing and as a response to the demands of the physical or social environment and the challenges of living. Without change normal life is impossible. Basic survival depends on it. The human ability to continue to have a fulfilled and varied life, adopting or discarding roles and occupations, changing relationships, developing interests and meeting challenges throughout all the stages of living is fundamentally dependent on being able to change.

Change may occur gradually, almost unnoticed, but often change is experienced as difficult, stressful, threatening or uncomfortable, especially when it is imposed by circumstances which appear beyond one's control, whether these are due to the changes of maturation and ageing or to external circumstances such as stressful life events including illness, bereavement, redundancy and divorce. Even pleasant events such as moving into a home of one's own, marriage, having children or being promoted require personal change.

When faced with stressful change the ability to cope or recover may depend on the degree to which the person can alter in response to these adverse circumstances. Someone who is fixed in rigid patterns of thought or behaviour can only react to things as they used to be, not as they now are. Such a person never manages to move away from loss, grief, physical limitation or personal disappointment. He is confined within limitations of his own making and by routines and habits which persist and are resistant to adaptation.

Every therapist rapidly becomes aware that the person who is positive, adaptive and flexible has a far better chance of living a fulfilling and satisfying life, even in the face of great difficulties or disabilities, compared to the non-adaptive person whose problems may be less challenging.

Occupational therapy is itself a process of 'changing through doing'. The principles of OT have been derived from the theoretical and scientific background of several of the fundamental processes of change, human development, human learning, and human adaptation.

As described in Chapter 3 these processes are hard to classify because they operate at various levels; each is large and complex enough to be described as a paradigm in its own right. They are also quite closely interlinked.

Studies of learning and development have given rise to much theory building and model making, with associated approaches. These have influenced the theories and practices of rehabilitation. As interpreted by various professions in education and health care, they have generated further AFRs and approaches. Adaptation has elements of all the other three, plus a strong influence from systems theory and from the practice of OT. Rehabilitation evolved as a synthesis of physical and psychosocial therapies aimed at achieving constructive change and recovery following illness or injury, and adapting to or compensating for the effects of residual disability.

Each of these processes has helped to influence and shape the philosophy and practice of OT and has been incorporated into the theory base of applied frames of reference and OT practice models.

Adaptation, in particular, is viewed as a central part of OT philosophy.

Adaptation is a change in function that promotes survival and self-actualization. Biological, psychological and environmental factors may interrupt the adaptation process at any time throughout the life cycle. Dysfunction may occur when adaptation is impaired. Purposeful activity facilitates the adaptive process. Occupational therapy is based on the belief that purposeful activity (occupation) including its interpersonal and environmental components, may be used to prevent and mediate dysfunction and to elicit maximum adaptation (American Association of Occupational Therapy 1995: statement of the philosophical base of OT).

Occupational therapy is concerned with the individual as a skilled and competent performer of a range of roles and occupations appropriate to his age, environment and culture; each process contributes in some way to the attainment and retention of skilled performance.

It is important for a therapist to identify which of these processes is most significant for her client. One cannot, for example, rehabilitate – restore – a skill which was never there to begin with; if the skill was not there it must be learnt. One cannot teach someone to use a skill if the prerequisite developmental potential is not present of if the required developmental level has not been attained. A person who cannot learn (attend to, perceive, store and recall information and relate this to his situation) cannot adapt. It is, therefore, important that the student understands the scope of these processes and their relationship to OT.

Summary: processes of change

- **Development**: produces change through maturation and by active use of innate abilities which build into complex skills.
- **Adaptation**: produces useful change which enables a person to respond to the demands of daily life and enhances and maintains health and well-being.
- **Rehabilitation**: is the intervention by the health care team which produces change which assists in the restoration of function and independence following illness or injury.
- **Education**: promotes learning which produces change through the acquisition of knowledge, skills, attitudes and values which are incorporated into daily life.

Q These four processes are widely used across the whole spectrum of OT practice. Probably you use one or more yourself or have seen them in use. With a colleague or in a small group, discuss the following questions using your own experience to provide illustrations.

1 Why is it useful to distinguish between the four processes?
2 From your current case load, select a patient whose main problem seems to fit one of the processes. How are you treating this person and how did you decide which approaches/techniques to use?
3 Would a different process give a new perspective on this person and his/her needs?
4 Do therapists make good use of educational theory? Explore some applications of different learning or teaching theories within your own practice.

THE PROCESS OF DEVELOPMENT

Development is usually described as a hierarchical process in which one stage has to be completed before the next. The first 18 or so years of human life follow a genetically programmed developmental sequence leading to maturation. Developmental stages are innate, and each person is born with a finite and predetermined package of potential. If the potential for performance is not there, nothing can be done about it; but the extent to which potential, however large or small, is turned into competent performance depends on environmental influences and opportunities to learn, discover, experiment, practise and gain experience.

The nature versus nurture debate remains unresolved. In the past decade environmental influences have been emphasized but recent studies comparing identical twins reared in differing environments suggest that genetic factors may be more important than previously thought, providing the potential for skills and, more controversially, even interests and preferences.

There does appear to be agreement that environment remains the most important factor; a person with the potential for genius would be profoundly limited if raised in an environment where there was a total absence of stimulation or conversation, whereas a person with severe learning difficulties would be able to make the best possible use of limited potential given individual attention and a richly stimulating environment.

Educationally, developmental theory is of use in looking at the way children learn and acquire skills (motor, perceptual, cognitive, social) (Piaget). In the context of adult learning, theories deal more with the sequence in which cognitive abilities and concepts are developed and refined (e.g. Bruner 1990).

Physiologically, developmental theories are concerned with the maturation of the central nervous system and the sequence of acquisition of neuromuscular control, proprioceptive discrimination and perceptual skills. Incomplete, retarded or dysfunctional development is very significant to the therapist since a person cannot perform in a manner for which he is developmentally unready.

Psychosocial developmental theories look at stages in the maturation of the individual's personality and self-concept.

Primary assumptions
- All individuals have developmental potential.
- The individual develops (physically, intellectually, emotionally, socially) in a defined sequence related to age.
- Stages in the developmental sequence cannot be missed or jumped if the individual is to function within the norms for his age/developmental level.
- The individual cannot function at a higher level than his stage of development. (But some authorities accept that it is possible to develop unevenly, and to be mature in some respects but not in others.)
- Environment, experience and opportunity limit or maximize the extent to which developmental potential can be fulfilled.
- Development is achieved by the integration of responses through practice, experiment and exploration; the therapist can facilitate development by reinforcing responses, aiding integration and creating the opportunities for practice and exploration (see Fig. 10.1).

Examples of associated approaches: Neurodevelopmental (Bobath 1990, Rood 1956; PNF;

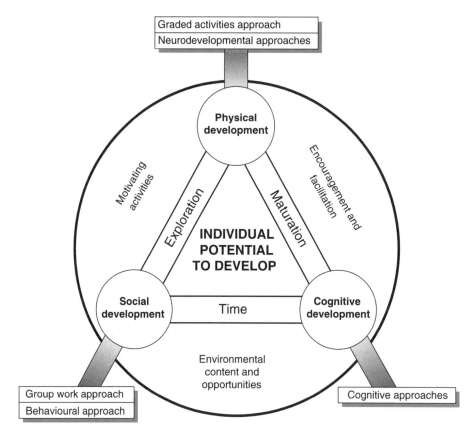

Figure 10.1 The process of development.

Conductive Education); cognitive disabilities (Allen); sensory integration (Ayres); spatiotemporal; facilitating growth and development (Llorens); development of adaptive skills; recapitulation of ontogenesis (Mosey).

Techniques: Those associated with the above approaches.

Criteria for evaluation of outcome: The individual has achieved the normal developmental level for his/her age/sex or has shown progression from one level to a more advanced one.

Advantages and disadvantages: The process of development is based on well-researched physiological, psychological and learning theories. Developmental approaches can benefit people with low abilities and severe learning deficits, as well as those who have regressed to a lower developmental level as a result of illness, trauma or stress.

Working developmentally can be slow and usually requires intensive therapy. The therapist must be confident and thoroughly competent when working neurodevelopmentally where effective application requires expert use of techniques which take practice and experience, and a sound comprehension of the basic theory. Progress can be retarded or lost unless all members of the team use the same techniques consistently. This model is not appropriate for deteriorating or terminal conditions (although some of the associated techniques may be) and may not be appropriate for elderly people.

THE PROCESS OF ADAPTATION

Adaptation is most important and influential process in the context of OT (Fig. 10.2). Schkade and Schultz (1992) have constructed a model

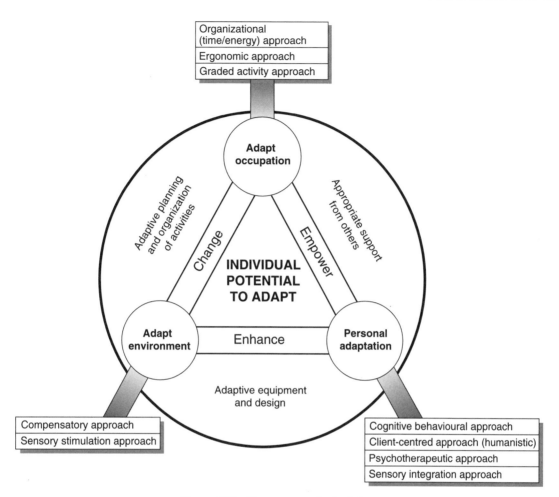

Figure 10.2 The process of adaptation.

based on adaptation and consider it to be 'of such significance that it functions as a paradigm within occupational therapy' (see Section 4).

Primary assumptions
- The ability to react adaptively to changing circumstances throughout life is essential for personal survival and well-being.
- Adaptation depends on the ability to perceive and respond to stimuli in the environment and to learn new responses when required.
- A person may be enabled to respond more adaptively by enhancing perceptual skills and interpretive ability, providing feedback for responses, promoting successful engagement in relevant occupations, developing problem-solving and planning skills, adapting tasks and environments to enhance performance.

In OT texts there are four distinct areas in which adaptation is discussed.

- Individual adaptation, a combination of physiological, perceptual and cognitive responses to the environment.
- Adaptive acquisition of skills, roles and occupations.
- Adaptations to occupations in order to facilitate performance.
- Adaptations to the environment to promote access and facilitate performance.

Of these, individual adaptation is the most important aspect. If the individual cannot adapt, learning new skills may be seen as irrelevant and alterations to tasks or environments are unlikely to be seen as useful or beneficial and are likely to be rejected.

Individual adaptation

Individual adaptation tends to focus on the relationship between what the environment demands and what the person does to meet those demands. The individual is seen as adapting when the person is able to organize data and make a response that meets the demands (Reed & Sanderson 1992).

Adaptation is essentially 'an active process of engaging the environment according to one's intentions' (Kielhofner 1992). It involves the person in exercising perceptual discrimination, and cognitive and sensorimotor control.

Adaptation is the active use of personal potential and learning opportunities in order to reach personal goals and to exert influence on the environment. Development, in a purely biological sense, is a finite process which is largely predetermined and ends when maturation is completed; but adaptation, like learning, can and should continue throughout an individual's lifetime.

One may fail to adapt because of faulty learning, but one may also learn a behaviour which is maladaptive, such as stealing or abusing drugs or alcohol. Seriously maladaptive behaviour is frequently associated with poor perceptions of personal control – the person either experiences his life as being controlled by others or by external circumstances, or he may seek to exert and impose personal control in maladaptive ways – through anger, bullying, abuse of another or by antisocial acts.

Humans are social beings who need to coexist with others within the boundaries accepted by a particular culture. Behaviour which is adaptive contributes to the individual's survival and well-being and to that of the society in which he lives. When an individual is adaptive he learns by his mistakes but then uses that learning in order to predict and avoid similar mistakes in future.

Behaviour which is maladaptive often fails to be predictive and either fails to meet the demands of the situation or actually makes the situation worse for the individual or someone else.

Adaptive behaviour should not, however, be equated with 'normal' behaviour (whatever that may be!), for slavishly following some perception of the norm, whether personal or cultural, may itself be maladaptive if what is required is change. Equally, behaviour which is idiosyncratic or even eccentric may sometimes be quite adaptive for the individual, even if society does not approve.

Adaptive acquisition of skills

Mosey describes a developmental frame of reference which she calls 'recapitulation of ontogenesis' (ontogenesis means change over time, therefore Mosey means 'repeating stages of development'). She goes on to describe this as being:

addressed to the development of adaptive skills … The term adaptive is used in the sense of being able to negotiate within the environment in such a way as to be able to satisfy one's own needs as well as those of others. It is used in the sense of creative use of the environment – not in the sense of conformity.

She lists six adaptive skills (see Ch. 9) (Mosey 1986).

An adaptive continuum has been proposed, starting with basic physiological homeostatic reactions, developing in turn adaptive responses (motor, sensory, cognitive, intrapersonal and interpersonal), adaptive skills and adaptive patterns (Reed 1984, adapted from Kleinman & Buckley 1982).

Kielhofner includes adaptation as an occupational performance skill, the components of which are: notices/responds (reacts to environment); accommodates (modifies actions or location of available objects); adjusts (makes some change to environment, introducing a new element); benefits ('anticipates and prevents undesirable circumstances from recurring or persisting') (Kielhofner 1995).

Enabling a person to adapt is a matter of finding a balance between the demands of the environment and the needs, wishes and abilities of the person. People may be inhibited from adapting because the environment is unsuitable or because they do not have the right skills or information. They may be inhibited by their attitudes, motivation, thoughts and feelings. People who do not perceive or interpret the environment correctly – because of physical, cognitive or psychological deficits – find it difficult to adapt because they cannot modify their responses appropriately.

Adaptation to occupations

As the individual moves from childhood through adult life to old age, it is necessary for him to be able to adapt and change the pattern of roles, occupations and activities at each stage. What is appropriate in childhood is usually not socially acceptable in adult life; the vigorous young adult requires a different pattern of engagement from that of the older person. New social roles – student, parent, pensioner – bring with them the need for different patterns to be developed.

Many people manage this process of adaptation naturally and without problems, but others find the changes difficult, especially at significant points such as adolescence, retirement or when coping with stressful life events – marriage, separation, childbirth, bereavement, loss of job or ill health.

People may need assistance to adapt what they do in a number of ways. Changes can be made to the pattern and balance of occupations, to the nature of the activity, its sequence, complexity or duration or to the tools and materials used.

Psychological or cognitive changes relating to occupations and activities may be even more important, e.g. moving from negative to more positive attitudes and patterns of thought, having expectations of success (or realistic judgement concerning likely failure) and setting achievable personal goals.

Successful participation in a variety of activities is seen as a means of promoting adaptation; the person may adapt by learning new skills, developing confidence and positive self-concept, and thus see himself as a competent performer who is capable of exercising a degree of control over his life.

Adaptation to the environment

The social environment may need changing so that people with whom the individual is connected give appropriate emotional support, cues or feedback to promote adaptive behaviour or provide practical help.

Changing the physical environment, as in helping a disabled person to choose home adaptations and arranging installation of these, is an important role for the therapist.

More subtle changes to the environment in terms of the level of stimulation and feedback it provides are also important in therapy and in certain learning situations.

Approaches: Adaptive techniques are included in a wide range of approaches, and in PEOP models.

Criteria for evaluation of outcome: The person is able to respond adaptively to the situations which confront her; well-being is enhanced; survival is promoted; the individual is able to function within socially accepted norms.

Advantages and disadvantages: Expresses many of the fundamental concepts and principles of OT and provides a practical framework for interventions which include the person, his occupations and environment.

The theory base is diffuse. Much is based on hypotheses and assumptions which need further research.

Theorists tend to make the assumption that an individual can always adapt, given the right assistance/environment, and do not take account of what to do when the individual appears incapable of change.

THE PROCESS OF REHABILITATION

Rehabilitation has been defined by the World Health Organization in 1974 as: 'the combined and coordinated use of medical, social, educational and vocational measures for training or retraining the individual to the highest possible level of functional ability'.

The overlap with education is plain; indeed, rehabilitation is sometimes called re-education. The root of the word is the Latin *habilitas*, meaning deftness or skill, so the word means literally, 'reskill'.

WHO further distinguishes between medical, social and vocational rehabilitation, as follows.

- **Medical rehabilitation**. The process of medical care aiming at developing the functional and psychological abilities of the individual and if necessary his compensatory mechanisms, so as to enable him to attain self-dependence and lead an active life.
- **Social rehabilitation**. That part of the rehabilitation process aimed at the integration or reintegration of a disabled person into society by helping him to adjust to the demands of family, community and occupation while reducing any economic or social burdens that may impede the total rehabilitation process.
- **Vocational rehabilitation**. The provision of those vocational services, e.g. vocational guidance, vocational training and selective placement, designed to enable a disabled person to secure and retain suitable employment.

In these definitions medical and social rehabilitation clearly involve an element of adaptation – the person needs to adjust to, and compensate for, his difficulties.

The process of rehabilitation requires a detailed knowledge of the client's medical, social and environmental circumstances; aims of treatment must be geared closely to the needs of the individual. Methods include use of techniques drawn from the biomechanical, neurodevelopmental, cognitive, behavioural, group work and, more recently, client-centred approaches.

As implied by the WHO definition, rehabilitation is viewed as an interdisciplinary process in which members of a team bring together skills appropriate to the needs of the client and work in close cooperation to achieve jointly agreed rehabilitative goals, normally under medical direction.

The aims of rehabilitation are well defined.

- To enable the individual to achieve independence in the areas of work and self-care.
- To restore the individual's functional ability to the previously attained level or as close to this as possible.
- To maximize and maintain the potential of retained, undamaged abilities.
- To compensate for residual disability by means of aids, appliances, orthoses or environmental adaptations.

Rehabilitation models

As discussed in Chapter 2 there has been an evolution of models of rehabilitation over the last two decades. In the UK rehabilitation is now a recognized medical specialism.

The biomedical model

The original model of rehabilitation is based on a linear, 'cause and effect' view of disability in which prescribed treatment is required to deal with the physical (or, in the case of mental illness, psychological) effects of an illness or injury.

Once the previous level of function has been attained or maximum improvement has been achieved, the patient is helped to resettle in the community and, if appropriate, to find employment. In this model the patient is expected to comply with the advice of the doctor and the rehabilitation team and to work actively towards his recovery in the manner suggested.

The strongest focuses of traditional rehabilitation are the restoration of physical abilities, including sensorimotor function, independence in activities of daily living, work skills and social skills.

The biopsychosocial model

This model was developed in recognition of the fact that disability is a much more complex problem than is suggested by the biomedical model. Treatment requires an integrated, holistic approach, dealing with physical, psychological, social and environmental aspects of the individual's situation.

In this model rehabilitation becomes a partnership between the individual, his family or carers, the rehabilitation team and official or voluntary agencies in the community.

The social model

This model goes further than the biopsychosocial model, regarding disability as a product of a failure of society to meet the needs of the individual. The emphasis is on normal living and full integration of every individual into society. Culture, social values and the design of the environment should be structured so that incapacity becomes virtually irrelevant and no longer prevents participation.

In this model the disabled individual is placed in the pivotal role of expressing his or her needs and obtaining from professionals and others the services which he or she wants and values.

Influences of rehabilitation models

The biopsychosocial and social models have now become dominant, and have influenced attitudes and widened the scope of practice. The new International Classification of Disease definitions of disability and its consequences (Glossary p. 167) clearly reflect this.

Reciprocally, it seems that the increasingly holistic approaches of rehabilitation professionals have also influenced theory building and the parameters of service delivery.

Approaches: As indicated in Fig. 10.3 a number of approaches are compatible with this model.

Examples of specific interventions
* Physical rehabilitation
  — assessment and retraining of activities of daily living
  — provision of aids and home adaptations
  — graded physical/cognitive/perceptual rehabilitation programmes (using biomechanical, cognitive or neurodevelopmental approaches)
  — specific prescription of remedial activities
  — work retraining and resettlement
  — prescription and provision of orthoses
  — prosthetic training
* Psychiatric rehabilitation
  — assessment of social and self-care skills
  — social skills training
  — behavioural modification
  — specific activities to redevelop cognitive, social, self-care or creative skills
  — industrial therapy, work retraining and resettlement
  — preparation for community living (group homes and hostels).

Criteria for evaluation of outcome: The lost function has been demonstrated to be restored to normal and/or a satisfactory method of compensating for residual disability has been found. The patient has been resettled in a normal, or adapted, domestic and/or work environment.

Advantages and disadvantages: This is a positive approach, aiming to improve necessary abilities, maximize existing function and compensate for deficits. Highly practical, it promotes problem solving, with a valuable, well understood team approach.

Because of its innately optimistic assumption of improvement, this process is less applicable to deteriorating, chronic or terminal conditions. It is also inapplicable in the context of learning disorders, since here it is a matter of 'habilitation', and the other processes are more appropriate. There may be a tendency to focus on the lost abilities, rather than on those which still exist. If application is allowed to become reductionist only the obvious problems may be tackled, perhaps dealing with effects rather than causes or failing to take account of psychological problems in a physical setting. Skills tend to be dealt with rather than roles or relationships. If overly prescriptive, the patient may be pressed to comply with action which is not his first choice. However, the fact that this model has stood the test of time better than most indicates that it has relatively few disadvantages.

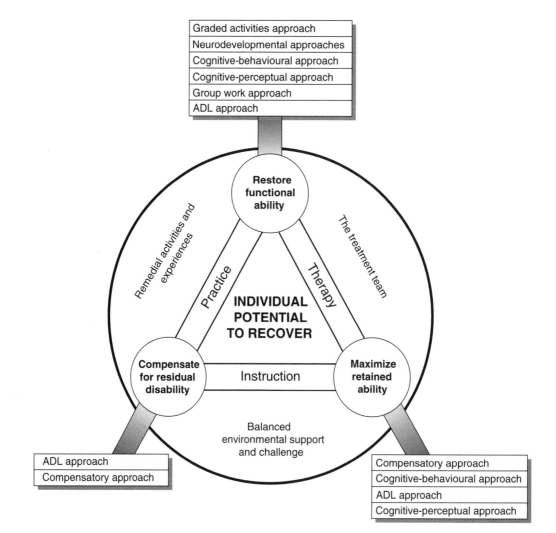

Figure 10.3 The process of rehabilitation.

THE PROCESS OF EDUCATION

Some therapists say firmly that occupational therapists are *therapists* not *teachers*. That is true, but it would clearly be misleading to say that therapists do not teach. Many spend much of their time doing so but often in an informal, unstructured manner, which may be so subliminal that both therapist and client fail to recognize the process. Mosey (1986) acknowledges that this has been so, but she has no doubts that 'the teaching–learning process has been a tool of occupational therapy since its inception'.

OT involvement in education can at other times be more formal and readily identifiable. Education of colleagues, other professions, health education for the general public, teaching specific skills, student education and supervision are important and integral parts of the therapist's role. Perhaps some of the misunderstandings arise from the fact that the therapist frequently teaches adults, a process which has been called *andragogy* (Knowles 1978) as distinct from pedagogy. Moreover, the therapist frequently deals with adults who have special learning needs. There has been considerable research into adult learning styles and appropriate methods of teaching adults, the more recent of which tend to emphasize the importance of moving towards student-centred and experiential styles of learning, rather than teacher-centred instruction. Except in the case of special needs or remedial teaching, where the edges between therapist and teacher truly blur, the therapist usually has a different basis for the use of educational techniques, and differing concerns from those of the teacher (Fig. 10.4).

Theories of learning and the related teaching techniques are derived from the primary frames of reference previously discussed.

- Physiological: researching into the neurophysiology of learning.
- Behavioural: breaking down complex behaviour into skills and subskills and viewing learning as a product of environmental reward and reinforcement.
- Cognitive: viewing learning as dependent on cognitive processes (remembering, processing, storing, retrieving) which then direct behaviour, and cognitive-developmental, looking at the sequences in which various skills are learnt.
- Social: seeing learning as linked to our perceptions of others and their behaviours.
- Humanistic: emphasizing that one cannot teach another person, only facilitate his experiential self-directed learning.

Primary assumptions
- Most human behaviour is learnt (but there are various theoretical explanations of the way in which this occurs).

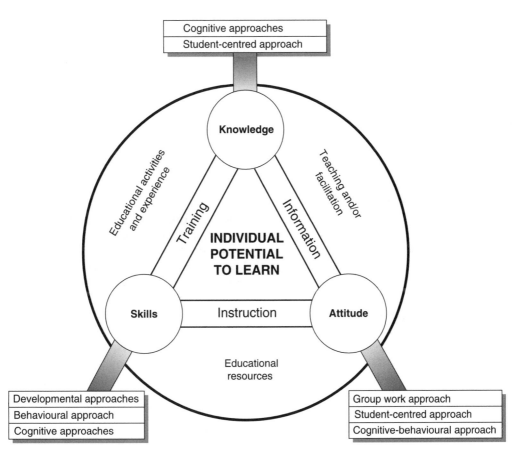

Figure 10.4 The process of education.

- Effective learning results in a long-lasting change in behaviour.
- It is possible to improve knowledge or skills or to develop attitudes by providing appropriate teaching, practice or experience.
- The context in which learning takes place can promote or inhibit learning.
- Given time and the right techniques, all but the most severely brain-damaged individuals are capable of some learning.

Examples of educational approaches: Physiological; behavioural; cognitive-perceptual; cognitive-behavioural; social; student-centred.

Examples of techniques

- Physiological, e.g. training motor skills and perceptual-motor skills; biofeedback.
- Behavioural, e.g. behavioural modification; errorless learning; chaining and backward chaining; habit training.
- Cognitive-perceptual, e.g. memory and perceptual training.
- Cognitive-behavioural, e.g. cognitive restructuring; anxiety management; assertion training.
- Cognitive-developmental, e.g. conductive education; portage.
- Social, e.g. social modelling; role-play; social skills training.
- Humanistic, e.g. student-centred learning; experiential learning.

Criteria for evaluating outcome: Learning objectives have been met. There is observed to be a permanent change in the individual's knowledge, skill or attitude as a result of new learning.

Advantages and disadvantages: Methods and contexts are so varied that a brief discussion of advantages and disadvantages is impossible. Possibly the main disadvantage is that any learning process takes time and learners experiencing difficulties require a large amount of individual attention if learning is to be effective.

THE DARE MODEL (DEVELOPMENT, ADAPTATION, REHABILITATION, EDUCATION)

An integrative approach

The DARE model is a description of a process rather than a set of theories. It is derived from a personal model of practice (Hagedorn 2000) which provides a means of using the OT process to integrate intervention using the processes of change which have previously been described. Although this model is not widely established, this description is included in the hope that it may assist therapists who prefer to take a process-driven approach to their work to do so in a more structured and coherent manner, rather than being somewhat vaguely holistic or eclectic.

It is a person-centred model and the focus is on competent occupational performance in the areas of self-care, leisure and work (the individual may define these for himself). It aims to enable and empower the person to cope as well as possible, given individual circumstances, with the activities which he wants or needs to do, to a necessary or satisfactory standard, whenever required, and to experience optimum quality of life.

It is described as a problem-based model because it seeks to use diagnostic reasoning to answer the question 'what is the problem?' by framing the problem situation in one or more of the following ways.

- **As a problem of development.** The person may have the potential to do more, but is unable to because he has not reached the developmental level necessary for functional performance. This may be because trauma has resulted in regression to a developmental level much lower than previously attained and not in balance with chronological age (e.g. following brain damage) or else that the person has for some reason (e.g. genetic, environmental) never reached the necessary developmental level (is not yet able, can't yet do). Since skills cannot be learned until the individual is developmentally ready, therapy must be aimed at developing potentials for performance until the necessary level is attained.

- **As a problem of adaptation.** The person is confronted by a situation which cannot fundamentally be changed and to which he has failed to adapt (e.g. a permanent disability or illness, a deteriorating condition, a set of challenging circumstances). In order to lead as full and satisfying a life as possible, adaptation must take place. Adaptation may be required to the environment, both social and physical, to the roles, occupations, activities and tasks which the individual wants and needs to perform, and the individual himself by making changes to his attitudes, values, thoughts, emotions or skills.

- **As a problem of rehabilitation.** The person was previously able to perform competently, but function has been lost as a result of illness or injury. In this case, therapy is aimed at restoring physical abilities or psychosocial skills as near as possible to the previous level by a graded programme of activity.

- **As a problem of education.** The person may be developmentally ready and able to perform, but has never learnt how to do so; he lacks the necessary skill, knowledge, appropriate attitude or experience. Alternatively, new circumstances may require that new learning takes place. In either case, intervention needs to be aimed at helping the person to learn what is needed in order to function competently.

Primary assumptions

- Performance problems can be analysed as being ones of development, education, rehabilitation or adaptation.
- Adequate data collection is essential for correct analysis of the problem.
- The individual's perceptions of his problem are central to the process of analysis.
- The apparent problem may not be the real one; the apparent solution may not be the best one. Some problems do not have solutions, but all problems respond to action within an appropriate process of change.

- In any problem situation there may be several applicable solutions – one should keep an open mind.
- Interventions should be directed towards goals which must be negotiated by client and therapist and defined before intervention begins.
- Progress should be monitored and action changed or the problem reassessed if results are ineffective.

Criteria for evaluation of outcome: The previously identified objective has been achieved and the identified problem is resolved.

Advantages and disadvantages: The use of this model (Fig. 10.5) represents a conscious attempt to view the person and his or her problems holistically and objectively before deciding on the nature of the problem and how (or if) to treat it. It places the person at the centre of this process and involves him closely in identifying and prioritizing problems in so far as this is possible for him. Each process is complementary to the others; it is possible to change the emphasis from one process to another during different parts of the intervention and to combine approaches from more than one process.

A wide range of relevant treatment techniques or approaches can be synthesized providing that techniques do not clash. It avoids the lack of focus which can arise if techniques are used eclectically in the absence of a coordinating model of practice, and also the danger of taking too narrow a view. Because it involves processes which are well understood by others, it is highly suitable for use in a multidisciplinary setting.

Use of this model can be adapted to most locations and specialities, although it is of especial use where a variety of types of problems are seen, e.g. in the community. It is suitable for all types of patients and can manage deteriorating or complex situations effectively. Promoting teamwork and providing measurable outcomes, the structured recording systems aid communication and evaluation.

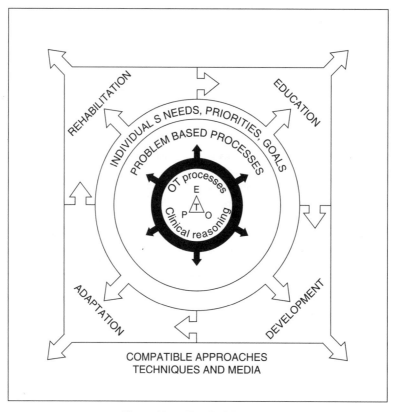

Figure 10.5   The DARE model.

There may be too much focus on negatives; strengths and assets may be ignored. The whole system relies on very accurate assessment and identification of the problem, and correct framing of it within one or more of the four processes of change. Incorrect evaluation, wrong priorities or poor solutions render intervention inappropriate or ineffective. It is not a uniquely OT model and may therefore lose its focus on occupational performance unless the therapist consciously maintains this. If the person-centred focus is lost it may become overly reductive or directive.

Person-environment-occupational performance models

11

INTRODUCTION TO PERSON-ENVIRONMENT-OCCUPATIONAL PERFORMANCE MODELS

In Chapter 3 we saw how concepts in OT have evolved from dependence on 'borrowed knowledge' to statements about the nature of occupational performance and the unique core principles or paradigm of the profession.

The first models to present these ideas were models of human occupation (e.g. Reed & Sanderson 1980, Kielhofner & Burke 1980). These attempted to explain the nature of human occupation and the dynamics and processes of occupational therapy and also sought to differentiate OT from other remedial or educative therapies.

In these models occupations are typically classified as work, leisure and self-care (or synonyms). The key components of human occupation are the person, engaging in an occupation within a specific environment.

As theorists continued to develop these ideas various models depicting the complex interactions between these three elements were proposed. The dimension of time, both developmentally and as it is used and structured during occupational performance, became important. The necessity of continued, adaptive occupational change and evolution throughout the life-span was also recognized.

By the mid 1990s there were numerous variations on these themes and a new generation of models evolved, initially referred to as 'occupational performance models', now also called person-environment-occupational performance (PEOP) models and person-performance-environment models (PPE). The initials PEOP will be used in this section.

Occupational science has provided a forum for research and publication, and there has been a reciprocal interchange of ideas concerning human occupation and occupational performance between occupational scientists and OT theorists (a number of prominent OT academics being both).

Whilst the literature produced by American theorists has been highly influential, it is significant that work has also been done in other countries, often by theorists who were working independently and generating very similar ideas without necessarily being aware at the time that other people were working on the same themes. Some of the models evolved during this period are shown in Table 11.1; there are others.

Despite individual differences in emphasis these models present a coherent view of OT and share common values and concepts, as described in Box 11.1.

COMMON VALUES AND BELIEFS EXPRESSED BY PEOP MODELS

These include:

- Belief in occupation as an essential part of human life, contributing to health and well-being
- Valuing the individual as unique and important, and respecting the individual's perceptions and wishes
- Considering that the subjective aspects of experience which contribute to personal meaning and quality of life are of fundamental importance.

A CONCERN WITH MEANING

Occupational therapists have always been concerned with both the functional and practical aspects of occupational performance and with creative activities which are not utilitarian.

It was realized at an early stage that people have emotional reactions to the things that they do, and that these reactions are closely bound up with motivation to perform. Affective reactions were, however, initially attributed more to the innate characteristics of the activity than to the internal dynamics of the individual's mind and personality.

The recent work done by PEOP theorists and by occupational scientists has focused attention on the individualized meanings which occupations have for their participants.

Box 11.1 Key features of PEOP models

The three key components of occupational performance are: the person, his or her occupations and the environment.

An occupation is a complex entity which places demands on the individual to acquire and use skills.

Occupations develop and change over time. Occupations also serve to structure and use time for the benefit of the individual.

Living involves a continual transaction or interaction between the person and the environment, which is mediated through the individual's occupations.

In order for optimal performance to occur there must be a good 'fit' between these components; that is, the person must have the required knowledge, skills and attitudes to perform the task, the task must be appropriate, contributing to health and well-being, and the demands of the environment must combine to optimize performance.

Humans function as open systems influenced by and influencing the environment. The abilities to learn new occupations and adapt occupational performance to meet new challenges are essential to health and well-being.

The content of the environment – physical, social and cultural aspects – produces a demand (or press) for an appropriate occupational reponse by the individual. The content of the environment can enhance or inhibit performance.

Occupational therapy aims to promote health and well-being through a client-centred process of engagement in occupations which are relevant to the individual.

Table 11.1   Person-environment-occupational performance models (dates refer to major publications: original presentation may be earlier)

Date	Country and theorist	Model title	Content	
1992	USA Reed & Sanderson	Human occupations model (3rd edn)	*Individual*	Skills: sensorimotor, cognitive, psychosocial
			Occupation	Productivity, leisure, self-maintenance
			Environment	Adaptation to and with environment
1992	CANADA Polatajko	Enablement model	*Individual*	Cognitive, affective and physical domains
			Occupation	Self-care, productivity, leisure
			Environmental dimensions	Physical, social and cultural
1992	UK Stewart	Model for the practice of OT	*Client*	Active participant in change
			Activity	The medium for change
			Environment	The context for change
			Therapist	Facilitates change
1995	USA Kielhofner	Model of human occupation (2nd edn)	*Human system*	Person interacting (input, throughout, output) with environment to produce occupational behaviour
			Environment	
			Task	
1997	CANADA Law et al	Person/environment/ occupation model: a transactive approach to occupational performance	*Person*	Unique being
			Environment	Variety of simultaneous roles: cultural, socio-economic, institutional, physical, social
			Occupation	Groups of self-directed functional tasks and activities
1997	USA Dunn, McClain Brown & Youngstrom	The ecology of human performance	*Person*	Ecology, or the transaction between person and context affects task performance which reciprocally affects the other elements
			Task performance context	
			Person-context-task	
			Transaction	
1997	USA Schkade & Schultz	Occupational adaptation model	*Person*	Occupations provide the means by which people adapt
			Interaction	
			Occupational	
			Environment	
1997	USA Christiansen & Baum	Person/environment/ occupational performance	*Person*	Performance results from complex interactions between person, occupations and environment
			Environment	
			Occupation	
1997	AUSTRALIA Chaparro & Ranka	Occupational performance model (Australia)	Eight interactive constructs: *Occupational performance Occupational roles Occupational performance areas Components of occupational performance (skills) Care elements of performance (mind, body, spirit) The performance environment Time Space*	These elements interact within time in each performance environment
1997	CANADA Canadian Association of Occupational Therapists	Canadian occupational performance model	*Individual*	Spiritual, physical, socio-cultural, mental
			Occupation	Productivity, leisure, self-care
			Environment	Social, cultural, physical
2000	UK Hagedorn	Competent Occupational Performance in the Environment (COPE)	*Person*	Person relates to therapist in the context of an occupation within environment
			Occupation	
			Therapist	
			Environment	Balance between the personal abilities, task demand and environmental demand required for competent performance

OT theorists are interested in meanings which are developed *empirically* through the experience of participation in occupations in a specific culture and context. Meanings are shaped by spirituality and by symbolic, transcendental, and ritual aspects of experience. Cultures develop shared meanings concerning particular occupations.

Meanings also arise as a result of intrapersonal dynamics concerning perceptions of self as an actor in the world, as expressed through personal narratives (Hasselkus & Rosa 1997). Whilst peak experiences inevitably carry a force of meaning, significant meanings may equally be derived from apparently mundane tasks and activities. Participation in meaningful occupations contributes to shaping personal identity (Christiansen 1999).

Recent academic papers, especially in the literature related to occupational science, discuss the meaning of occupation and its relevance in OT (e.g. Trombley 1995b, Wilcock 1999a,b).

The concern with personal meanings has led to an interest in spirituality and its impact on individuals' lives and their reactions to therapy, an area which was not formerly given much attention (e.g. Do Rozzario 1994, Collins 1998, Rose 1999, Hume 1999). The Canadian Occupational Performance Model (Townsend 1997) emphasizes the importance of spirituality.

TIME

What we do takes place in the stream of time within which we live our lives. This may seem obvious: however, the importance of the interactions between what we do and the lived experience of time is only just being recognized within OT literature and research.

Our tasks, activities, occupations and roles change over time (*occupational ontogenesis*). What we do also structures our use of time and gives meaning to it.

Observing and analysing occupational performance within different episodes of time may provide us with information about the nature of tasks, the ways in which they nest and enfold, and the ways in which skills evolve and are used.

ADAPTATION

Another strong theme is the need for humans to make adaptive responses. Occupations need to change over time as the individual takes on new roles or meets new challenges in her life. As described in Section 3, failure to adapt fast enough, or with sufficient flexibility and innovation, results in occupational dysfunction.

OCCUPATIONAL DYSFUNCTION IN PEOP MODELS

Occupational dysfunction stems from either an imbalance between the demands that occupations and environments place on the individual and that person's ability to react, adapt to and meet these demands, or deficits in the person's environment or occupations, or a combination of these things (Box 11.2). Occupational dysfunction adversely affects well-being.

PEOP MODELS DESCRIBED IN THIS SECTION

The following PEOP models are summarized (dates indicate main publications):

- Activities Health (Cynkin & Robinson 1990)
- Model of Human Occupation (Reed & Sanderson 1992)
- Model of Human Occupation (Kielhofner 1995)
- Occupational Adaptation Model (Schkade & Schultz 1992)
- Enabling Occupation (CAOT 1997)
- Competent Occupational Performance in the Environment (COPE) (Hagedorn 2000).

The models are presented in approximate chronological order. They each provide a different view of the same basic concepts. Most of these models have been produced by individuals or collaborating OT academics. The exception is the Canadian model, which has been

---

Box 11.2   Occupational dysfunction in PEOP models

Occupational dysfunction includes:

Occupational deprivation	The individual is prevented from engaging in a full and satisfying repertoire of occupations.
Occupational alienation	The individual suffers from a sense that his occupations lack meaning and satisfaction.
Occupational imbalance	The individual has a narrow range of occupations and engages in one aspect of life to the exclusion of others.

Specific problems contribute to these dysfunctions, including:

Participation problems	The individual cannot do the things he wants and needs to do.
Resource problems	The individual cannot gain access to the resources he needs. The environment either fails to provide (*afford*) them or there are barriers which impede access.
Temporal problems	Tasks take longer to perform; the individual finds it difficult to plan and sequence performance and fails to use time effectively.
Relationship problems	Difficulties arise in constructing and maintaining a network of social support and personal relationships appropriate to the individual's age and culture, which help to sustain roles and occupations.
Problems with occupational identity	The individual has a negative image of self as an effective actor within his or her life; this results in self-fulfilling prophesies of failure, and inability to make adaptive responses to correct this.
Problems with role identity	The individual either lacks a sense of having valued roles, or adopts one role to the exclusion of others.

---

produced over a period of time by a national OT association.

HOW DO OCCUPATIONAL PERFORMANCE MODELS CHANGE THE NATURE OF INTERVENTION?

A PEOP model acts as a primary filter which serves to ensure that the therapist considers all three sides of the occupational performance triangle and delivers a holistic, client-centred service which is demonstrably 'pure OT' and not something else.

The models are based on the biopsychosocial or social models of disability and place emphasis on promoting 'wellness' in occupational terms, rather than dealing with 'illness'.

Some models are theory driven; the model alters how the therapist will perceive the client, and provides a set of assessments designed for use within the model. Other models in this family are process driven and provide a structured version of the OT process to aid clinical reasoning.

It must be said, however, that the links between the assessment process used to identify need within the parameters and language of the model, and subsequent actions by the therapist, are not always made explicit. It appears in most cases that, having used the model initially, the therapist then reverts to a compatible applied frame of reference, modified by the PEOP model, to provide an approach to structure the details of therapy (Fig. 11.1). Use of a PEOP model may lead to the exclusion of some applied frames of reference if they appear incompatible with the philosophy of the model.

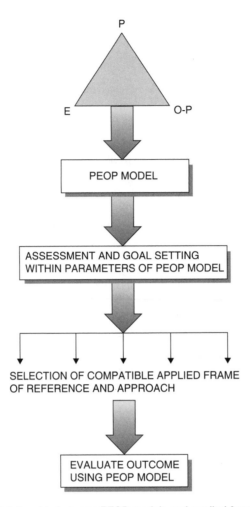

Figure 11.1   Relationship between PEOP models and applied frames of reference.

12

PERSON-ENVIRONMENT-OCCUPATIONAL PERFORMANCE MODELS

ACTIVITIES HEALTH MODEL

Simme Cynkin and Anne Mazur Robinson

Origins

This model was originally developed by Simme Cynkin in the 1980s in the USA. It was later presented in a more evolved form (Cynkin & Robinson 1990) together with a student-centred, experiential activities-based curriculum for OT education.

Like most American models produced during this period, it owes a debt to Mary Reilly's work on occupational performance. It differs from other models in focusing on activities rather than occupations and describing participants as actors.

The biosocial model adopts a strongly client-centred approach, emphasizing the idiosyncratic nature of experience and the personal meanings and emotions which activities evoke (Fig. 12.1).

It is not a model which is widely known or used in the UK and it is included in this section principally because it offers a provoking discussion of the richness of human participation in activities, and the ways in which the therapist can respond to this richness and use it as a means of therapy.

Assumptions about activities

Cynkin explores a number of assumptions which are keys to the concept of activities health. These are based on theories derived from behavioural, cognitive, educational and social psychology and sociology.

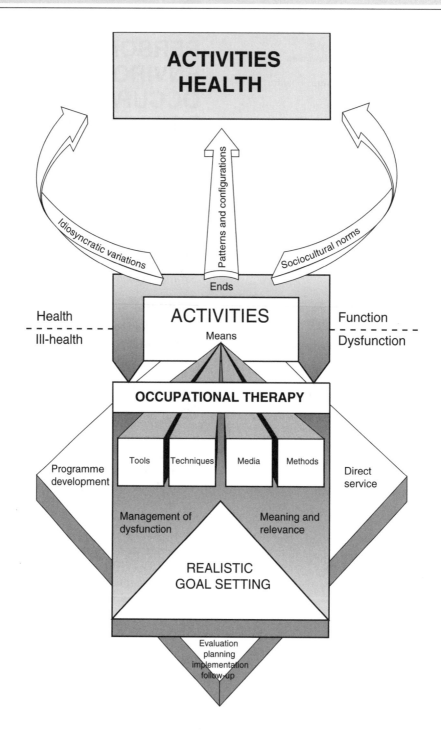

Figure 12.1 The activities health model (after Fig. 5.1 in *Occupational Therapy and Activities Health* by Cynkin, (1990) with permission. Published by Little, Brown and Company).

- Activities of many kinds are characteristic of and define a human existence.
- Activities are socioculturally regulated by a system of cultures, beliefs and customs and are thus defined by and in turn define acceptable norms of behaviour.
- Change in activities-related behaviour can move in a direction from dysfunctional to functional.
- Change in activities-related behaviour from dysfunctional to functional takes place through motor, cognitive and social learning (Cynkin & Robinson 1990).

Challenges to occupational taxonomies

Cynkin criticizes the usual work/leisure/self-care division as too restrictive and points out that perception of role and the nature of participation is highly individual. Sociobiological and sociocultural classifications are proposed as alternatives.

Activities health

This is defined as follows:

a state of well-being in which the individual is able to carry out the activities of daily living with satisfaction and comfort, in patterns and configurations that reflect sociocultural norms and idiosyncratic variation in number, variety, balance and context of activities.

Occupational therapy and activities health

Activities, to foster health, require the following of the actor: the use of the hands; conscious problem solving; creative activity.

Cynkin explores the ways in which activities of daily living are 'both ends and means in the practice of occupational therapy'. Activities engage the actor in a very special way: by performing an activity you become increasingly the thing you are trying to be – taking on the roles, skills, culture, meanings of the activity. (A similar concept is also developed by Kielhofner 1995.)

Therefore, through engagement in systematically selected activities, function can be developed and restored.

Activities analysis within this model includes far more than the usual skills-based format. It involves having an appreciation of the historical and cultural significance of each activity, and its subjective and phenomenological aspects – symbolism, personal meanings, personal preferences and style, feelings, effects of environment.

A version of the usual occupational therapy process is used to structure therapy.

Examples of applications: A wide selection of physical, developmental and psychiatric case studies are given implying widely applicable use with a wide age range.

Examples of approaches: Therapy must be activity based and the graded activities approach and educational approaches are predominant. However, these may be employed from biomechanical, neurodevelopmental, cognitive-behavioural, cognitive-perceptual or projective (psychotherapeutic) perspectives; the compensatory approach may be used. Little reference seems to be made to group work and analytical theories do not appear to have much place in this model.

Outcome measures: The authors provide an Idiosyncratic Activities Configuration questionnaire (Cynkin & Robinson 1990) which is intended for student use but could be adapted for use with a client. Guidelines for a Work Interview are also provided.

Other outcome measures and assessments are not discussed.

Critique

This is an early version of an occupational performance model, which differs in several respects from the mainstream versions. Notably, it challenges some of the ideas concerning the classification of occupations and avoids the use of the word 'occupation' in favour of 'activities'. This may well have lost the authors some support from theorists who prefer the accepted terminology, but it does belong to the PEOP family.

The presentation of the model (Cynkin & Robinson 1990) is intended as a guide to student-centred learning, rather than as a text on use with clients, although case histories are given.

The value of the model lies in the authors' deep understanding of the subjective nature of engagement in activities, and the link between activities and health. It is as much a statement of philosophy as it is of practice.

The authors also place much emphasis on activity analysis and the applied use of activities. They describe one-to-one therapy rather than work in groups.

It is rather less clear how assessment is to be conducted or how the model relates to other approaches. Whilst the theoretical research base is explored there is not much evidence of outcomes in practice. This model is seldom referred to in other texts and it is not clear whether it has become widely influential. It is included principally because it presents a valuable insight into aspects of human occupation and the therapeutic use of activities.

HUMAN OCCUPATIONS MODEL

Kathlyn Reed and Sharon Sanderson

Origins

This model has evolved over some 20 or more years, and is based on Reilly's work on occupational performance. It was first presented in 1980 in *Concepts of Occupational Therapy* by Kathleen Reed and Sharon Sanderson. This account is based on the 3rd edition, which was published in 1992 with some material from a summary of the model presented by Reed (1984).

Unlike Kielhofner's version, the model is process driven, but it shares with the model of human occupation a focus on occupations as fundamental to human existence and health. Reed and Sanderson use a version of the human occupations model which depicts the individual as possessing sensorimotor, cognitive and psychosocial (formerly intrapersonal and interpersonal) skills, engaging in productivity, leisure and self-maintenance, and aiming for adaptation to and with the environment (Fig. 12.2).

The model is based strongly on the processes of development, learning and adapting. Participation in occupations and alterations of the environment are both seen as powerful mechanisms for change. The approach has become increasingly client centred. It is problem based, and considers problems as being grouped in four areas: biological, psychological, social and occupational. Of these the occupational element is central; the other areas overlap, giving rise to biosocial, psychosocial and biopsychological aspects.

Reed and Sanderson are particularly concerned to identify the unique processes, concepts, techniques, concerns, assumptions and outcomes of OT. They focus on 'wellness', not the medical model which is concerned with 'illness'. Their view of the process and application of OT is highly structured. It is stressed that occupations can be therapeutic because they are the natural vehicles for normal development and adaptation and for the primary learning of skills. Skill assessment, development and retraining is seen as a main concern of occupational therapists. The OT can help the individual to develop adaptive responses through participation in occupations.

The key concepts of the model are discussed in detail and then expressed as a series of assumptions which underlie the practice of OT. Some of the key statements are summarized below.

Details of OT 'service programs', i.e. the services which OTs can provide in various specialities, are given, management aspects are explored, and there is a comprehensive glossary. This model is relatively accessible and has been quite widely adopted. It also forms one of the foundations for the development of the Canadian model of human occupation which will be described later.

Key assumptions

Assumptions about a human being

- **A person is:** a biopsychosocial and spiritual being; a unified whole; an open system energy unit; the sum total of the individual's life experience.

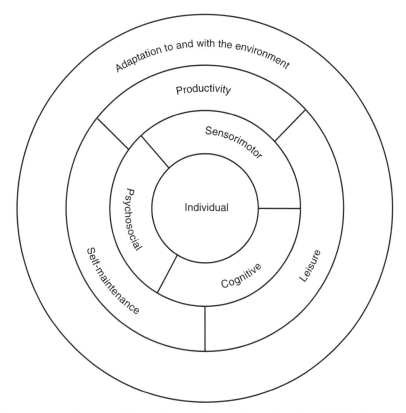

Figure 12.2   The human occupations model (reproduced with permission from Reed (1992) *Concepts of Occupational Therapy*. Copyright held by Williams and Wilkins).

- **A person has:**   the capacity for thought and sensation; needs; responsibilities; potential; basic rights.

Assumptions about occupational performance

These include statements concerning the central role of occupations in enabling the individual to continually change and adapt, meet responsibilities and change the environment, and the importance of occupations in maintaining health and a satisfying life. Occupations are determined by and occur in response to environmental factors.

Assumptions about occupational dysfunction

Dysfunction occurs when changes (ill health; injury; ageing; environment; etc.) affect the ability to use knowledge, skills or attitudes to adapt or adjust through the use of occupations.

Assumptions about health

Health is a total condition which is dynamic and changing. Illness affects occupational performance in several ways, including the reduction of energy, disruption of patterns and changing the person's abilities to perform occupations.

Assumptions about humanistic health care

These are philosophical statements concerning the person, the professional, the meaning of illness and the practice of health care which are difficult to summarize without losing their essence. The general thrust is optimistic and holistic, as expressed by the final statement 'both the person receiving care and the professional are whole human beings interacting in the healing effort'.

Assumptions about receiving health care services

These are statements of patient rights and expectations.

Assumptions about delivering health care through occupational therapy

These statements concern the aims of OT which should enable the client to:

- Achieve the highest level of occupational performance and adaptive behaviour consistent with the client's goal
- Return to a normal living environment in the community if possible
- Increase independent, adaptive behaviour and decrease dependent, maladaptive or non-adaptive behaviour
- Increase successful occupational performance and decrease non-productive occupational performance.

Health care programmes in occupational therapy are classified as:

- Prevention
- Developmental
- Remedial
- Environmental adjustment
- Maintenance.

Assumptions about occupational therapy

The benefits of active doing in terms of promoting occupational performance and improving or restoring skills are described:

Therapy (in occupational therapy) is the use of directed, purposeful occupations to influence positively a person's sense of well-being and, thus, the state of a person's health.

Therapeutic occupations: These should be one or more of the following: meaningful; purposeful; goal directed; challenging. Reed offers an extended discussion of the individual and subjective nature of meaning in terms of occupational performance, and emphasizes the essentially purposeful nature of therapeutic activities (Reed 1984).

Assumptions about the therapeutic use of occupations

These statements summarize the rationale for the use of occupations as therapy.

The environment: Reed and Sanderson propose that occupational performance is influenced by the environmental context and content which may enhance or impede learning and performance. They suggest that analysis of the environment by the therapist is a significant therapeutic tool in identifying the causes of maladaptation and in enhancing and facilitating adaptive performance. The environment can be subdivided into:

- Physical environment: inanimate, non-human and natural aspects
- Psychobiological environments: the individual self – the human being
- Societal cultural environment: people and their cultures, attitudes, values and means of organization.

Occupations: These can be divided contextually into:

- Self-maintenance
- Productivity
- Leisure.

Also into component *tasks* (but each occupation is performed as a gestalt).

Occupations have three *performance areas*. Each performance area requires the use of abilities and *skills* which are classified as:

- Sensorimotor
- Cognitive
- Psychosocial

  — psychological (formerly intrapersonal)
  — social (formerly interpersonal).

Each of these skills is subdivided and defined.

The performance of occupations requires three *general elements* which are learnt:

- Knowledge
- Abilities
- Attitudes/values.

In her 1984 summary of the model Reed also describes three *specific elements* related to occupational therapy:

- Orientation: to time, place and person
- Order: pattern and direction
- Activation: ability to move and think.

Occupational adaptation and adjustment: The goal of the individual is life satisfaction through occupational adaptation. Occupations should enable the person to relate to the environment and to meet their needs by balanced performance within the areas of productivity, self-maintenance and leisure. Occupations have associated standards, roles and meaning for the individual. Occupational behaviour is either adaptive or mal/non-adaptive.

- Adaptive behaviour: uses skills to achieve balanced experience of occupations consistent with social norms and self-satisfaction.
- Maladaptive behaviour: is unsuccessful, and/or unacceptable to the individual or society.
- Non-adaptive behaviour: fails to produce an effective results, but is not unacceptable.
- Occupational dysfunction: involves problems in planning and/or performing an occupation; or in evaluating feedback of results.

Outcomes: In her 1984 summary of the model Reed states outcomes of OT clearly and concisely and these are best quoted as written.

- The person will be able to perform or have performed those occupations which meet the individual's needs and are acceptable to the person and society.
- The person will have the necessary performance skills which compose the occupations in the individual's repertoire of self-maintenance, productivity and leisure.
- The person will have a balance of occupations such that actualization, autonomy and

achievement are attained to a maximum degree of adaptation.
- The person will be able to adapt to the environment or cause the environment to adapt to the individual.
- The person will be able to meet both deficiency needs and growth needs.
- Where the person is unable to perform skills independently, assistive devices or equipment or other environmental adjustments may be used (Reed 1984).

Applications: Any person who, for whatever cause:

- has failed to develop occupational skills in any of the three areas
- has temporary or permanent loss of occupational skills
- whose performance of occupational skills will require non-routine modification
- is at risk of losing occupational skills (Reed & Sanderson 1980).

Approaches: Any holistic approach appropriate to the problem. Cognitive-behavioural techniques may be appropriate, and neurodevelopmental and biomechanical ones are certainly suggested. Analytical techniques seem less relevant since they are not compatible with a strongly humanistic approach and the model does not pay much attention to unconscious mechanisms.

Outcome measures: Assessment is related to observation of functional performance of self-care, work and leisure occupations and use of specific skills – sensorimotor, cognitive and psychosocial.

Both formal and informal methods are suggested, but the authors do not specify assessments. There do not appear to be any assessments developed for use within the model, and outcome measures are not discussed.

Critique

This is a process-based model which is structured around the usual procedures of OT. The model takes a biopsychosocial perspective emphasizing 'wellness' rather than 'illness'. It explores the unique contribution of OT and provides a practical, problem-based approach to intervention.

The theoretical basis is less evolved than that of other models. Whilst this makes it more accessible to practitioners it may make it less convincing from an academic standpoint. The description of practice appears somewhat physically biased.

MODEL OF HUMAN OCCUPATION

Gary Kielhofner

Origins

The model of human occupation (MOHO) was first published in the *American Journal of Occupational Therapy* by Gary Kielhofner in collaboration with others (Kielhofner & Burke 1980; Kielhofner 1980a, b; Kielhofner et al 1980). He started the conceptualization which led to the model in the mid 1970s. These ideas were developed in his book about the model (Kielhofner 1985) and restated in a second edition (Kielhofner 1995) with some changes. The model has been seminal and has provoked an interest in model building and professional philosophy.

Kielhofner has drawn together a number of different areas of knowledge and a basic familiarity with these theories and their terminology is helpful. These include systems theory, cognitive psychology, developmental psychology, humanistic psychology and social psychology (including the theory of symbolic interactionism). Of these systems, theory is of fundamental importance, and a summary of this will be given shortly.

The OT roots of the model stem from Mary Reilly, a respected American OT theorist whose work during the 1960s and 1970s has been highly influential. Reilly developed a hypothesis expressing the central belief of OT as follows: 'that man, through the use of his hands as they are energized by mind and will, can influence the state of his own health' (Miller & Walker 1993).

She developed the paradigm (or model) of occupational behaviour based on four concepts: 'the human need to be competent and to achieve;

the developmental aspects of work and play; the nature of occupational role; the relationship of health and human adaptation' (Miller & Walker 1993), and went on to develop the concept of a work–play continuum and devoted much time to the study of the importance of play in human life. Reilly also became interested in open systems theory whilst developing her ideas.

Kielhofner was one of Reilly's students, and his thinking has clearly been strongly influenced by her work.

Key assumptions

- The human organism can be described as an open system.
- Occupations are central to human experience, survival and satisfaction.
- Occupational areas of work, self-care and play (leisure) evolve and change throughout the individual's life.
- Occupational performance results from the interaction of three sub-systems: volition, habituation and mind-body-brain performance subsystems.
- People seek to explore and master their environments. Environment affords opportunities and presses for performance.
- The individual's perceptions of feedback from the environment are crucial in directing further output of adaptive occupational performance.

The human open system

Kielhofner summarizes the main idea behind open systems theory as follows:

living phenomena are dynamic self-organizing entities exhibiting ongoing interaction with their environments (unless stated otherwise quotations are taken from Kielhofner 1995).

The dynamic aspect of this theory relates to flows of energy within the system; when new energy reaches a kind of critical mass, 'whole new states of organization emerge spontaneously'. He also states that 'components of a dynamical system behave in ways that cannot be predicted by their individual properties'.

The concepts of energy and organization are important. Because the human being is an open system, behaviour is influenced by the interactions of the human system, the task and the environment, and by the information which the environment and the task contribute to the situation. Kielhofner describes this as 'the "ballet" of ordinary occupational behaviour'. Behaviour is fluid and improvisational, 'spontaneously organized in real time and in the context of action'.

Kielhofner's ideas about the ways in which the human system is able to change adaptively include the following concepts.

- That new behaviour becomes established by repetition – by continually acting as a musician or cook or football player the person gradually *becomes* it. Equally, if such behaviour is discontinued, the associated roles and skills also fade.
- That change can be produced by alterations within the organization of the internal system or by changes external to it.
- That change can sometimes be dramatic and produces a whole new organization in a short space of time.
- Sometimes a small change in some significant factor can be the key to large changes in behaviour.
- The human system continually changes and adapts: 'the organization at any point in time is a reflection of the dynamic process of life'.

Internal organization of the human system

An open system operates by a process of circularity into, through and out of it.

Output, or the product of the system, is occupational behaviour which is classified as work, daily living tasks, leisure or play. Output is either adaptive or maladaptive (functional or dysfunctional).

Input (intake) to the system comes from the environment; it includes information from the surrounding people, events and objects.

Throughput processes input, organizes information, makes predictions on which to

base action, and decisions on further action or output.

Feedback returns information to the system about the performance and consequences of action both from input and from monitoring of internal processes, e.g. how one feels about what one has done.

The three subsystems can be summarized as:

Volitional subsystem = will. The mechanisms whereby we choose what to do.

Habituation subsystem = roles and rules. The basic cognitive structures with which we organize our lives.

Mind-body-brain performance subsystem = skills. The means by which we carry out occupational behaviour.

Subsystems of the model of human occupation (Fig. 12.3)

Volitional subsystem

'System of dispositions and self-knowledge that predisposes and enables persons to anticipate, choose, experience and interpret occupational behaviour.'

Volitional structure: 'Stable pattern of dispositions (cognitive/emotive orientations towards occupations) and self-knowledge (awareness of

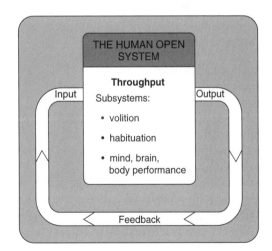

Figure 12.3 The model of human occupation (reproduced with permission from Creek J (1990) *Occupational Therapy and Mental Health*. Churchill Livingstone, Edinburgh).

self as actor in the world) generated from and sustained by experience.'

Three areas of volitional structure
- Personal causation (knowledge of capacity: awareness of abilities; sense of efficacy: perception of control)
- Values (personal convictions; sense of obligation)
- Interests (attraction: enjoying certain activities; preference: enjoying certain ways of doing things).

Volitional process
- Attending (attention; anticipation; reacting to possibilities)
- Experiencing (finding occupations enjoyable; feeling more or less able)
- Choosing (occupational and activity choices).

Volitional narratives: This is based on the ideas of Mattingly (Mattingly & Fleming 1994) concerning the role of personal 'story-telling' as used by people to make sense of their lives (see narrative reasoning).

Habituation subsystem

'An internal organization of information that disposes the system to exhibit recurrent patterns of behaviour.' The operation of the habituation system involves processes and systems described in cognitive psychology.

Habituation structure:
- Habit (acquired by repetitions; operates at a preconscious level to influence behaviour; habits involve cognitive processes)
- Habit map (guides the perception of familiar events and related action)
- Internalized roles (awareness of social identity with related obligations, situations and behaviour)
- Role scripts (understanding of social situations and expected responses)
- Influence of habits on occupational behaviour
- Influence of roles on occupational behaviour.

Habituation process: The organization of the subsystem guides immediate responses and also change over time. Principles include:
- Habit formation and change (habits: preserve patterns of behaviour; resist change; may outlive their usefulness)
- Socialization and role change (formal and informal roles change and need to be renegotiated throughout life).

The mind-body-brain performance subsystem

'Refers to the organization of physical and mental constituents which together make up the capacity for occupational performance.'

Constituents of the performance subsystem:
- Musculoskeletal system
- Neurological system
- Cardiopulmonary system
- Symbolic images (guide the system in producing behaviour).

The components of the subsystem receive, organize and process information in order to plan action and effect performance.

Kielhofner discusses the above subsystems at some length, and also explores environmental influences on occupational behaviour and the development of occupation. Occupational dysfunction is defined and explored within the terms and concepts of the model, together with methods for gathering data and the principles of therapeutic intervention. Considerable work on application has been carried out in the past 10 years and since this discussion is detailed and can only be appreciated in the original text, where case examples are given, no attempt will be made to summarize it here.

Much work has also been done to develop assessment tools for use within the model. These include the Occupational Case Analysis Interview (OCAIRS: Kaplan & Kielhofner 1989) and various checklists for role participation, personal interests, and self-rating of strengths and weaknesses (examples and cases are given in Kielhofner 1995).

One development resulting from the model has been research into skill in occupational

Table 12.1   Motor and process skills

Motor skills	Process skills	Communication/ interaction skills	Social interaction skills
Posture	Energy	Physicality	Acknowledging
Mobility	Knowledge	Language	Sending
Coordination	Temporal organization	Relationships	Timing
			Coordinating
Strength and effect	Organizing space and objects	Information exchange	
Energy	Adaptation		

Adapted from Kielhofner (1995)

performance. The taxonomy of skills is summarized in Table 12.1. Each skill has an associated list of actions.

This research into skills has resulted in the production of a detailed assessment instrument, the Assessment of Motor and Process Skills (AMPS). The assessment depends on very precise observations of the use of the listed actions in the context of functional performance. In order to use this, the therapist requires special training to become an accredited user. Development and research continue and this work may well have implications for use beyond the confines of the model of human occupation.

The influence of environment

Kielhofner stresses the importance of the effect of the environment on the individual. He describes 'press' – the demands which an environment places on an individual for appropriate occupational behaviours. The environment contains things which are capable of arousing us and promoting action – objects, tasks, social groups, cultural pressures. A degree of novelty and stimulation is pleasurable and promotes exploration and mastery. People generally perform well in such conditions.

Too much press, e.g. excessive novelty, overstimulation, and being bombarded by the demands of an environment, results in stress, anxiety, uncertainty, helplessness, frustration, anger, overarousal and inability to cope (flight or fight responses). People fail to perform in such environments. Too little press results in apathy, withdrawal and disinterest, in which circumstances people also fail to perform well.

A continuum of function and dysfunction

In his earlier publications Kielhofner described a continuum stretching from expert function to total dysfunction. Functional occupational behaviour is achieved through *exploration* ('curious investigation in a safe environment to discover potentials for action and properties of the environment') which leads to *competence* ('striving to be adequate to the demands of a situation') and *achievement* ('striving to maintain and enhance standards of performance').

Dysfunction runs from *inefficiency* ('reduction or interference with performance resulting in dissatisfaction') to *incompetence* ('inability to routinely and adequately perform') and finally *helplessness* ('total or near-total disruption of performance').

In restoring function the client may need to be taken through the stages of safe exploration until competence is achieved, and will then need to experience competent behaviour over a period of time in order to gain a sense of achievement.

Occupational narratives: Kielhofner and his associates have become interested in the techniques of using narrative as a means of understanding occupational 'life-stories', and uncovering personal meanings (Helfrich & Kielhofner 1994).

Outcome measures: Since the model has now been in use for some 20 years it has been possible for academics and practitioners to collaborate in the production of a comprehensive set of assessment tools.

These are available as manuals, and some also have training videos.

The assessments available at the time of writing are:

The Assessment of Motor and Process Skills (AMPS) (Fisher 1994) The user requires training and accreditation to use this assessment.

The Assessment of Communication and Interaction Skills (ACIS) (version 4.00) (Forsyth et al 1998)

The Worker Role Interview (version 9) (Velozo et al 1998)

Work Environment Impact Scale (WEIS) (version 2.00) (Moore-Corner et al 1998)

Volitional Questionnaire (VQ) (version 3) (de las Heras et al 1998)

Occupational Self-Assessment (version 1.00) (Baron et al 1998)

Occupational Performance History Interview (version 2.00) (OPHI2) (Kielhofner et al 1998).

Compatible approaches. Any holistic approach may be used with this model and also biomechanical and neurodevelopmental approaches used in physical rehabilitation. Classic behaviorist and psychoanalytical approaches do not appear compatible.

Critique

As one of the longest established models in this group MOHO has been refined and developed into a highly coherent presentation of theory and practice. It is widely used in USA and elsewhere with a variety of clients in physical rehabilitation and mental health settings. There is an extensive literature and research is continuing.

Criticisms have been made on practical and philosophical grounds. The underlying conceptualization, especially the use of systems theory, is quite complex and not always readily accessible, although recent presentations have attempted to simplify these ideas. Use of the evaluative process does seem to imply that a reasonable length of time is available for exploration of all the issues. This may not always be available. There is a somewhat weak link in the presentation of the model between its use to diagnose and frame performance problems and the subsequent selection of an approach to direct further action.

OCCUPATIONAL ADAPTATION MODEL

Janette K Schkade and Sally Schultz

Origins

The model was generated by academics at the Texas Women's University, where in 1989 the concept of occupational adaptation was selected as the basis for doctorate study.

The authors have researched the background to their assumptions and hypotheses with care, and the original sources are comprehensively referenced. They draw extensively on the work of OT theorists, and other researchers with an interest in the dynamics of adaptation.

This model integrates the concepts of occupation and adaptation. It has been influential in theory building and is frequently cited.

Key assumptions

The fundamental assumption is that humans, when faced with environmental or internal challenges, are able to adapt their occupational responses in order to meet these new demands (Fig. 12.4).

The authors restate their assumptions in a simplified format (Schkade & Schultz 1998) as follows.

Competence in occupational performance is a lifelong process of adaptation to internal and external performance demands.

These demands occur naturally within occupational roles and within the context of person–occupational environment interactions.

Dysfunction occurs when there is disruption of the adaptation process.

The adaptation process can be disrupted by impairment, disability or handicapping conditions as well as stressful life events.

The focus of intervention is to maximize the individual's internal adaptation process.

Improvement in occupational performance is dependent on improvement in the adaptation process.

Further key assumptions are reprinted as stated in Schkade and Shultz (1992) with minor editing.

Occupation provides the means by which human beings adapt to changing needs and conditions and the desire to participate in occupation is the intrinsic

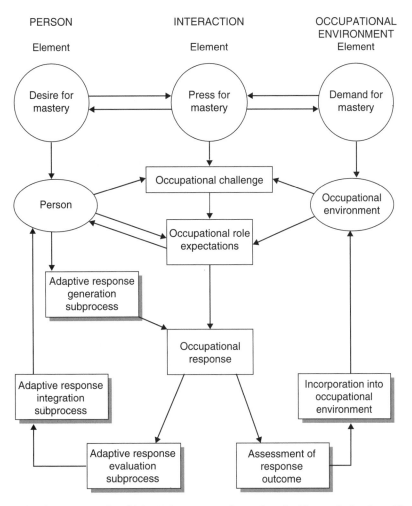

Figure 12.4   Schematic of the occupational adaptation process (reproduced with permission from Fig. 1 in *Occupational adaptation: Toward a holistic approach for contemporary practice*, part 1, by Schultz S & Schkade JK 1992. Copyright held by the American Occupational Therapy Association, Inc).

motivational force leading to adaptation. People desire to behave adaptively and masterfully.

The three basic elements of the occupational adaptation process are the person, the occupational environment and the interaction of the two as they come together in occupation.

The person is made up of three systems: sensorimotor, cognitive and psychosocial. All three systems are present and active (to varying degrees) in every occupational response.

All three systems are required for successful occupational adaptation.

The person's state of occupational functioning is the cumulative effect of that person's occupational process activity.

Occupational adaptation is a normative process that is most pronounced in periods of transition, both large and small. The greater the adaptive transitional needs, the greater the importance of the occupational adaptation process, and the greater the likelihood that the process will be disrupted.

Dynamics of occupational adaptation

In their original papers Schkade and Schultz make a number of proposals concerning the way in which occupational adaptation occurs. These are based on physiological and cognitive theories, and the reader needs to refer to the original text to understand these ideas. The key points may be summarized as follows.

- People have characteristic *adaptive response modes:* that is, they develop persistent, habitual patterns of occupational behaviour (*homeostasis*). These are likely to continue to be produced until some internal or external change demands revision. The individual is then challenged to change behaviours and acquire new patterns (*occupational adaptation*).
- When assessing performance the therapist can distinguish between adaptive response modes which are stable (*primitive*), changing (unstable or *transitional*) or an effective blend of stable and unstable responses (*mature*).
- A flexible response, in which a lot of new patterns are tested and tried, is more likely to produce adaptive change; the behaviour then needs to be stabilized and becomes part of a new pattern of performance. If appropriate and effective new response modes fail to be acquired a state of *occupational dysadaptation* develops.

This hypothesis is linked to the concept that we each have a finite supply of *adaptation energy*. This powers our ability to make adaptive changes. It is sufficient to meet the demands of normal living, but very stressful circumstances may deplete or overwhelm the available supply. Successful occupational adaptation requires that the supply of adaptation energy be used judiciously and to best effect.

Adaptation takes place by means of three cognitive *adaptation subprocesses*. These are:

- *The adaptive response generation subprocess*
- *The adaptive response evaluation subprocess*
- *The adaptive response integration subprocess*.

These subprocesses are complex constructs. Put simply, the *generation* subprocess creates a plan of action and unifies skills from the three domains to produce an integrated response. The *evaluation* process observes and weighs up the results, in terms of efficiency, effectiveness, satisfaction and personal mastery. The *integration* process assimilates the new

response into the repertoire of daily occupational behaviours.

A detailed discussion of the processes of adaptation by the same authors is provided in Christiansen & Baum (1997) and readers are advised to refer to this.

Terminology

The key terms are defined (Schkade & Schultz 1992) as follows.

Occupations are activities characterized by three properties: active participation, meaning to the person, and a product that is the output of process. The product may be tangible or intangible. Occupations include work, play, leisure and self-care (with physical, social and cultural subsystems).

Adaptation is a change in the functional state of the person as a result of movement towards relative mastery over occupational challenges.

Occupational adaptation (the state) is a state of competency in occupational functioning towards which human beings aspire. It is also a *process* through which the person and the occupational environment interact when the person is faced with an occupational challenge calling for an occupational response reflecting an experience of relative mastery.

Relative mastery is the extent to which the person experiences the occupational response as efficient (use of time and energy), effective (production of desired result) and satisfying to self and society.

Implementation of the model

In their second article (Schultz & Schkade 1992), the authors propose an holistic approach, grounded in meaningful occupation.

They suggest that 'The most beneficial effects of occupational therapy may occur when the occupational therapist focuses on the internal workings of the patient's occupational adaptation process.' This view is strongly restated in their later summaries (1997, 1998).

In order to achieve this, the therapist must address the priorities valued by the patient and provide a facilitating therapeutic climate offering experiences which foster occupational adaptation.

This model may be regarded as theory driven, since the concepts and terms of the model determine how the client is assessed and the way in which the problem is described. The following questions are listed as a guide to data gathering and assessment (Schultz & Schkade 1992).

What are the patient's *occupational environments and roles*? Which role is of primary concern to patient and family?

What occupational performance is expected in the primary *occupational environment and role*?

What are the *physical, social and cultural* features of the primary occupational environment and role?

What is the patient's *sensorimotor, cognitive and psychosocial status*?

What is the patient's level of *relative mastery* in the primary *occupational environment and role*?

What is facilitating or limiting *relative mastery* in the primary *occupational environment and role*?

Following assessment and identification of areas of dysadaptation, the therapist will plan how to help the client to understand personal occupational responses and achieve occupational adaptation.

This may be done in two ways, by promoting *occupational readiness* or by *occupational activity*.

Compatible frames of reference

The authors do not explicitly describe supporting applied frames of reference. Their approach is indicated by analysis of the cases which are used as examples.

When developing *occupational readiness* (that is, improving basic skills in the sensori-motor, cognitive and psychosocial systems) the authors appear to favour traditional techniques of physical, cognitive or neurological rehabilitation.

However, the statement that therapists should focus on 'internal workings of the patient's occupational adaptation process' (1992) and guide clients to a greater understanding of these processes, might support the use of a cognitive-behavioural approach.

Occupational activity 'engages the client in tasks that are part of the occupational role selected by the client' (1998). The authors stress the benefit of the spontaneous experience of occupation as a meaningful whole, and engagement in novel and/or creative activities which involve

integrative processing and problem solving, so reductionist approaches are not compatible.

Outcome evaluation: Evaluation is framed within the terms of the model. The following questions are suggested (1992).

How is the program affecting the patient's *occupational adaptation process*?

Which *energy level* is used most often (*primary or secondary*)?

What *adaptive response mode* is used most often (*pre-existing, modified or new*)?

What is the most common *adaptive response behaviour* (*primitive, transitional or mature*)?

What outcomes does the patient show that reflect change in the *occupational adaptation process*? Self-initiated adaptations? Enhanced *relative mastery*?

Generalization to novel activities? (Is there improvement in efficiency, effectiveness and satisfaction of self or others?)

What program changes are needed to provide maximum opportunity for *occupational adaptation* to occur?

Critique

The synthesis of the concepts of occupation and adaptation within the occupational performance framework is valuable. The model strongly states the fundamental importance of adaptation and outlines the mechanisms by which this might take place.

The extent to which this model is used in practice, and the links between theory and the details of subsequent intervention are unclear. Judging from the literature the model has been used in both clinical and community settings. It is reported to be the subject of continuing research.

There are no published assessments specifically associated with this model, but the structured approach to enquiry and evaluation is clearly set out.

The complexity of some of the concepts concerning the dynamics of adaptation and the use of specific terms to describe this may be inhibiting at first sight. The student is advised to read both the original papers and subsequent presentations. A practitioner would probably need to review some of the background material given in the references in order to understand the concepts fully.

ENABLING OCCUPATION: THE CANADIAN MODEL OF OCCUPATIONAL PERFORMANCE

Canadian Association of Occupational Therapists

Origins

The model evolved as a result of a joint initiative between the Canadian Association of Occupational Therapists (CAOT) and the Canadian Department of National Health and Welfare.

This began as an attempt to provide clear guidelines for OT practice, incorporating material which could be used to set standards and promote quality assurance. A principal objective was to develop an outcome measure for occupational therapy.

The task group reviewed the literature on OT theoretical and philosophical concepts, collected and criticized numerous assessments, produced a report (Department of National Health and Welfare & CAOT 1983) and engaged in wide-ranging dialogue within the profession. Further reports were produced (Department of National Health and Welfare & CAOT 1986, 1987).

As a result of this work the Canadian Occupational Performance Measure (COPM) manual (Law et al 1994) was published. The COPM has been under development for several years, and is well researched. Comprehensive references are given in the COPM manual and in *Enabling Occupation*. Additional work has been published in journals.

Having produced the Guidelines and COPM, the CAOT task group found that they had inevitably become engaged in building a conceptual foundation for practice: the Guidelines were developed into a model, *Enabling Occupation* (CAOT 1997) (Fig. 12.5).

This model provides a very clear account of the core concepts and values of OT, and a process for client-centred service delivery.

Key assumptions

The model is based on a set of values and beliefs concerning: occupation, the person, the

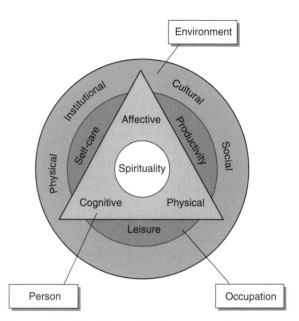

Figure 12.5 Canadian model of occupational performance (reproduced with permission of CAOT Publications from *Enabling occupation: An occupational therapy perspective*, 1997, Fig. 1).

environment, health and client-centred practice. The central goal of OT is to enable clients to engage in occupation.

Occupations, classified as leisure, productivity and self-care, are of fundamental importance to human beings. They have practical and economic functions enabling people to meet their health and survival needs and to structure and manage their environments. Occupations also provide sources of purpose, meaning, choice and control in human lives.

The environment has cultural, institutional, physical and social elements. These elements combine to impact on the individual, affecting the nature and scope of occupations. The environment also provides the context within which occupational therapists practise.

The person is viewed as an integrated being having cognitive, physical and affective skills and a dimension of spirituality. The latter dimension is 'the essence of self ... because people are spiritual beings, each individual is appreciated as a unique person'. The authors accept that 'whilst for some people spirituality is a religious vision, for others ... it is a feeling or sense of meaning'. Spirituality is seen as the driving force of self-determination and choice.

The model adopts a developmental perspective on the individual. The person changes over time, and occupations also evolve over time in relation to life events and the challenges of the environment.

A central construct in this model is the conviction that the client must undertake the process of determining need and planning action; the therapist's role is to enable this process.

Enabling: This defined as:

processes of facilitating, guiding, coaching, educating, prompting, listening, reflecting, encouraging or otherwise collaborating with people so that individuals, groups, agencies or organizations have the means and opportunities to participate in shaping their own lives.

The guidelines deal explicitly with issues of choice, risk and responsibility in client-centred practice. It is accepted that the process of therapy may entail risk taking, and that clients need support to enable success and, at times, to cope with the experience of failure. Perhaps more controversial is the bold statement that the therapist should 'facilitate clients to choose outcomes that they define as meaningful even if the occupational therapist does not agree'.

The occupational performance process

The model is process driven, and a seven-stage version of the occupational therapy process is described.

- Name, validate and prioritize occupational performance issues (using COPM).
- Select theoretical approaches.
- Identify occupational performance components and environmental conditions.
- Identify strengths and resources available to client and therapist.
- Negotiate targeted outcomes; develop action plan.
- Implement plans through occupation.
- Evaluate occupational performance outcomes.

Intervention: Enabling occupation allows for a flexible range of interventions, applicable to a wide range of physical, psychosocial or environmental problems. A selection of case examples describing the application of the model is provided.

Service provision to the client is also set within the context of the service environment and the wider context of society as a whole.

Outcome measures: The initial assessment is conducted using the client-centred Canadian Occupational Performance Measure (COPM) (Law et al 1994). By means of this the client is enabled to identify 'problem' areas of performance which are of personal concern and to rate them for difficulty and satisfaction with performance. The tasks are then put into priority order, and an action plan is developed to deal with the issues. The COPM also provides an outcome measure when performance is eventually re-evaluated by the client and the initial and final rating scores are compared.

Additional assessments may be used if required, provided that they are compatible with a client-directed approach.

Compatible approaches: It is possible to use various approaches, selected on the basis of the client's problem(s). Physical rehabilitative, psycho-emotional, neuro-integrative, socio-adaptive, developmental and environmental theories of occupational function and dysfunction are suggested. If further assessment is required any suitable, well-constructed assessment drawn from an accepted frame of reference can be used to provide further information. Use of such supplementary assessments might, however, have to be modified to be compatible with the strongly client-centred approach to evaluation.

Critique

This model is unique in having been constructed by a national OT association over a period of years. It is therefore coherent in presentation and refreshingly free of over-complex jargon and elaborate concepts. It provides a well-structured and practical guide to service delivery, with an in-built mechanism for evaluation of outcomes. It is subject to continuing research and evaluation.

The adoption of a highly client-centred approach may, however, produce problems in cases where the client is not readily able to determine goals. The process of facilitating goal planning could be lengthy, and the acceptance by the therapist of client goals 'come what may', whilst a logical consequence of the adoption of a true client-centred approach, may not always be practical or desirable.

COMPETENT OCCUPATIONAL PERFORMANCE IN THE ENVIRONMENT (COPE)

Rosemary Hagedorn

Origins

COPE is a person-centred, process-driven, occupational performance model which includes the concept of a hierarchy of occupational levels.

I developed this model between 1995 and 2000 as a means of making explicit connections between the hypotheses and assumptions which underpin the dynamics of OT and the core skills used by the therapist (see Hagedorn 1995a, 1995b, 1997, 2000).

The basic concepts were influenced by reading the work on occupational performance by Kielhofner, Reed, and other American theorists. Obvious similarities with the work of other theorists will be noted: however, in 1995, when the concepts were beginning to be formulated I had not encountered the work of the Canadian or Australian theorists, and was intrigued to discover subsequently that many of our ideas had obviously been developing in parallel and from similar roots. The model is included as a British contribution to the field.

Key assumptions

Competent, adaptive occupational performance is essential to human health and well-being.

Occupational performance is complex. It can be understood as an intentional, productive process which takes place when a person is doing a task, in a specific environment, within a definable time frame. Performances occur at different levels, determined by the time frame and the nature of what is being done.

Humans acquire knowledge and synthesize skills from the domains of action, interaction and reaction to perform tasks.

Performance of tasks places a demand on the individual to learn, adapt and respond. The process of performance and perceptions of the consequent product create changes within the individual. As a result of this intrinsic linkage the occupational therapist can use tasks as effective media in promoting adaptation, encouraging learning, improving health and enhancing well-being.

Competent, adaptive performance depends on a balance between the performance demands generated by the task and the environment and the ability of the person to respond to these. If the balance between these components is disturbed performance will fail to occur or may be ineffective. Dysfunction is viewed as a consequence of the loss of a successful and balanced relationship between these elements.

Adaptive change can be facilitated by employing the processes of development, adaptation, rehabilitation and education (see Section 3).

Because occupational analysis is a key to the evaluation of both performance problems and remedial action, it is proposed that the therapist should use a structured approach to analysis and intervention. This is based on identification of the occupational level at which dysfunction is occurring. Three occupational levels are described. The level is defined by the developmental and organizational complexity of what is being done and the duration of the time frame. The environment is also conceptualized as having levels or zones defined by proximity to the user (Table 12.2).

Application

The model provides a conceptual framework for OT, and also a practical technique for systematic exploration and identification of the causes of dysfunction (Hagedorn 2000) (Fig. 12.6).

Table 12.2   COPE: occupational and environmental levels

Occupational level	Time frame	Type of performance	Environmental level
Developmental		Actions Interactions	
Proto-occupational	Up to 1 minute	Reactions Performance units	Immediate environment
Acquistional *Constructive*	Up to 3 minutes Up to 10 minutes	Task stages Tasks	
Effective	Up to 1 hour	Tasks Activities Routines	Near environment
	Longer time frame not exceeding 1 day	Activities Routines	Used environment Exploratory area
Organizational	Several days or weeks	Occupations Roles	
	Months or years		

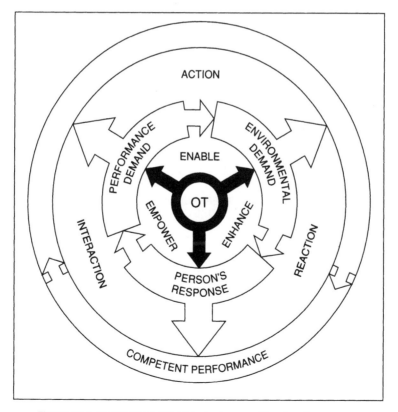

Figure 12.6 Occupational therapy and occupational performance.

The therapist can intervene to restore balance or fit and to promote competence by working with the individual to achieve adaptive change or by altering elements in the environment or by changing occupations or aspects of the way a task is structured and performed.

Core processes

In order to provide intervention the therapist uses four core processes in combination:

- Therapeutic use of self
- Assessment of individual potential and needs
- Analysis and adaptation of occupations
- Analysis and adaptation of environments.

Occupational therapy

Occupational therapy takes place when the therapist 'enters the occupational performance triangle' (Fig. 12.8) and works with the person in the context of a specific portion of an occupation in a particular environment for a defined, mutually agreed purpose.

A problem-based, process-driven approach is used to work with the client to discover the origin of the performance difficulty or deficit. This may be due to an external factor originating in the task or environment or to an internal problem affecting the individual's ability to respond to demand, which stems from a developmental deficit, acquired impairment, educational need or need for adaptive change.

The six stages in this process are worked through in a collaborative partnership with the client.

Making a profile of the client: as a past, present and future performer of roles and occupations in the environment(s) which the client uses; forming some consequent assumptions about

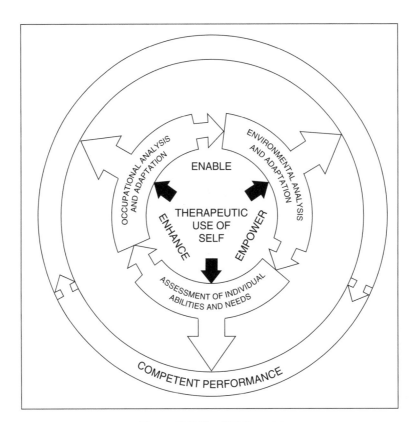

Figure 12.7 The COPE model.

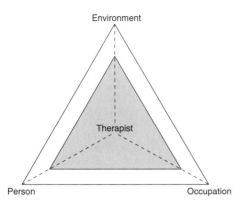

Figure 12.8 Person-occupation-environment-therapist triangle.

the nature of the situation and the relevance of OT.

Naming the problem: specifying the areas of concern to the client, and any deficits in occupational competence.

Diagnosis: framing the problem: analyse the nature of the problem using the PEO triangle (as affecting the client, the task or the environment or a combination of these). If the difficulty originates with the client, decide which process of change (development, adaptation, rehabilitation, education) is appropriate. Select an applicable AFR. Conduct further assessments if required. If the problem originates with the task or the environment, outline the type of action required.

Prioritize: decide what is to be done, and what should be done first, taking account of practical considerations and available resources.

Action plan: work with the client to explore alternative solutions and actions and agree goals and an outline plan.

Review: evaluate results and end intervention or adapt action plan as required.

It is recognized that some clients may not find it easy to identify or formulate personal goals and that guidance from the therapist is legitimate in the early stages of intevention in order to facilitate action.

Outcome measures: Any well-structured assessment may be used. At the lowest occupational level specific measures can be used. As the performance being assessed moves upwards through the levels, a wide range of functional assessments can be used provided that these are employed within a client-centred approach (see Hagedorn 2000 for lists of assessments).

Critique

The model attempts to provide a practical, structured, problem-based approach to OT. It gives the therapist a simple visual representation of the model which aims to provide an understandable rationale for what OT may achieve. COPE ensures that the therapist remains focused on key issues and skills. The approach is flexible; the therapist may move from being relatively directive to being totally client centred, according to the situation and in response to client progress.

Although based on accepted hypotheses and assumptions, the model has not been independently evaluated or researched, and, being a recent model, it is not widely used. There is no related set of assessments although any client-centred, well-validated tool can be used initially and subsequent assessments can be drawn from the selected frame of reference.

EXPANDED DEFINITIONS AND GENERAL GLOSSARY

Note

The Glossary includes words defined in the text, and words used in connection with models and professional practice. It does not include medical or psychological terms which may readily be found in specialist dictionaries, but a few terms which may be difficult to find or are notoriously confusing are defined. Where there are two meanings, or where several differing definitions exist, the alternatives are given.

Sources for definitions

Proliferating definitions are of no use to the student or to the profession. Where clear definitions exist which are compatible with the text, I have used these, and sources are indicated as shown in the code below. Those marked (RH) are my own.

(At)   Atkinson et al 1993 Introduction to psychology,
            11th edn. Harcourt Brace Jovanovich

(Cr)   Creek J (ed) 1990 Occupational therapy and mental
            health: principles, skills and practice. Churchill
            Livingstone, Edinburgh

(WS)   Hopkins H L, Smith H D (eds) 1988 Willard and
            Spackman's occupational therapy, 7th edn.
            Lippincott, Philadelphia

(Kh)   Kielhofner G 1992 Conceptual foundations of
            occupational therapy. F A Davis, Philadelphia

(Kh95)   Kielhofner G 1995 A model of human occupation ·
            theory and application. Williams and Wilkins,
            Baltimore

(Lov)   Lovell R B 1987 Adult learning. Croom Helm,
            London

(Polgar)   Polgar S, Thomas S A 1991 Introduction to research
            in the health sciences, 2nd edn. Churchill
            Livingstone, Edinburgh

(R)   Reed K L, Sanderson S R 1992 Concepts of
            occupational therapy, 3rd edn. Williams and
            Wilkins, Baltimore

(COD)   Sykes J B (ed) 1982 The concise Oxford dictionary,
            7th edn. Clarendon Press, Oxford

( )   *Other authors given in brackets.*

PHILOSOPHICAL TERMS

(Note: quotations come from Honderich 1995)

Atomism Educationally, a view that knowledge is constructed of numerous small parts which may be learnt separately or sequentially (as opposed to learning holistically). In philosophy, atomism involves making very simple factual statements which may build more complex understandings.

Causality A relationship in which something follows directly from the preceding thing or event. Philosophers discuss the nature of 'causes', argue over their effects and develop complex laws of causation.

Determinism A doctrine that human action is not freely chosen but is decided by external forces acting on the will.

Dualism A theory which recognizes that mind and matter are two separate things. There are various dualist theories. 'Substance dualism holds that the mind or soul is a separate non-physical entity, and that the soul might be able to exist apart from the body.' Property dualism accepts the division but not the possibility of independent existence of the mind/soul.

Empiricism Is 'a view which bases our knowledge, or the materials from which it is constructed, on experience through the traditional five senses'. In science, *logical empiricism* holds that all scientific claims must be evaluated on the basis of empirical evidence. In OT the word is used rather loosely to indicate knowledge or skill developed through practical experience.

Epistemology Is 'the branch of philosophy which is concerned with the nature of knowledge, its possibility, scope and general basis'. Epistemologists explore the nature of belief and fact, discuss the degree to which we can know anything for certain (scepticism), study the sources of knowledge (sensation, memory, introspection and reason), and construct theories of meaning and learning.

Existentialism A set of (usually very complex) ideas concerning the nature of human existence, individuality and consciousness of self. *Angst* is the sense of unease or concern about one's self and one's existence from which we all suffer in the course of the struggle to become an individual. Sartre's views on the central importance of *choice* in human life, and Heidegger's concept of *authenticity* have been influential in humanistic psychotherapy.

Free will The belief that humans have the capacity to make reasoned choices (as opposed to them being decided for us). This doctrine is complex and is related to arguments about the degree to which we can be held morally responsible. *Libertarians* believe that 'despite what has happened in the past, and given the present state of affairs and ourselves just as we are, we can choose or decide differently than we do – act so as to make the future different'.

Gestalt Originally a psychological theory concerning perception, gestaltists see the world as consisting of wholes which hold together and are irreducible, losing meaning if broken into parts.

Holism 'Any view according to which properties of individual elements in a complex are taken to be determined by relations they bear to other elements.' Holism is the opposite to atomism or reductionism. In OT it relates to an ecological systems view of the individual who can only be understood in relation to his total environment, previous life history, occupations and current circumstances.

Humanism 'The tendency to emphasize man/woman and his/her status, importance, powers, achievements, interests or authority.'

Humanistic psychology Is concerned with the uniqueness of the individual and explores subjective experiences and values. Various person-centred educational and psychotherapeutic approaches have been developed along humanistic lines. (Humanistic medicine has a similar basis.)

Logical positivism A development from *positivism*, this movement was originally concerned with a logical system for verifying the truth, or falsity, of written statements. It has become attached to later ideas concerning scientific enquiry being based on the systematic verification of data.

Meaning Meaning is an attribute of information or a situation which gives it significance and importance and enables the individual to 'make sense' of it. Philosophers have attempted to understand 'the meaning of meaning' using various approaches: linguistic, perceptual, cognitive and epistemological.

Mechanism Mechanists believe that humans operate like machines, having parts which combine to produce relatively fixed effects or products or that cognitively the mind operates as a 'supercomputer'.

Monism Is usually taken to mean that the mind and body are one and inseparable. (Other monist theories concern the singular nature of substances.)

Phenomena Things which can be perceived by our senses (contrasted with *noumena*, things which can be understood through abstract reasoning).

Phenomenology An important philosophical movement, originally a theory of knowledge. Phenomenologists are concerned with understanding consciousness and the sense of self, uncovering the *essences* of things, through both direct and indirect knowledge and a process called *eidetic reflection*. In OT the term tends to be used to indicate an holistic approach which takes account of the personal perceptions of the individual.

Philosophy Seeking after wisdom or knowledge, especially that which deals with ultimate reality or the most general causes and principles of things and ideas and human perception and knowledge of them (COD). There are numerous philosophical schools of thought and special areas of enquiry, including *epistemology* and *metaphysics*, the study of ultimate reality and existence.

Postmodernism A general movement in the arts and philosophy in the late 20th century which tends to favour pluralism and rejects the idea of any single 'truth' or finite view of an event. Postmodernists may attempt to deconstruct and challenge accepted ideas in order to reinterpret them on a broader basis.

Rationalism A view that knowledge should be based on reason not on sensory experiences which may be fallible.

Reductionism In science, reductionists 'attempt to make explanations in terms of ever more minute entities'. In OT reductionism is usually used to indicate the opposite view to holism, that is, of sytematically breaking a problem, situation or thing into its smallest constituents, without reference to the overall context.

TERMS USED TO DESCRIBE THEORY AND ITS PRACTICAL APPLICATION IN OCCUPATIONAL THERAPY

Approach

Ways and means of putting theory into practice; the practical application of a model or frame of reference, including style of relationship, assessment method, use of special techniques.

Assumption

An assumption is a statement which you accept as true and on which you base your actions. We need to make assumptions because we cannot found action on a continually changing set of 'ifs, buts and might bes'. Occupational therapy is based on a set of assumptions about the occupational nature of human beings and the ways in which engagement in occupation may be therapeutic. Whilst these ideas are generally accepted by occupational therapists they need to be viewed critically. An assumption may be soundly based on theory or merely a kind of working hypothesis. An assumption may or may not be correct. (One should try to be careful to distinguish between theories, hypotheses and assumptions, although this can be difficult.)

Clinical reasoning

The cognitive processes used by the therapist when evaluating information, making decisions, naming and framing problems, setting goals and deciding on action concerning the client. Clinical reasoning may result in the selection of a model or frame of reference or be guided by a previously selected approach.

Concept

In psychology a concept is defined as 'the properties or relationships common to a class of objects or ideas' (At). Concepts can be expressed in words (or by a symbolic representation). For example, to understand 'occupational therapy' one must first have concepts of 'therapy', 'occupation', 'person' and so forth.

Concept is often used as a synonym for 'idea'. Thus, 'conceptal foundations for practice' or 'concepts of occupational therapy' are the related ideas which build theories which define the basic concerns of the profession.

Fact

A fact is a true proposition (Honderich 1995). A scientific fact is one which is based on objective research which has proved the proposition to be correct. Unfortunately, the simple view that 'a fact is true' is deceptive. It depends on the kind of fact one is describing, and the philosophical standpoint of the person who is describing it. Thus, whilst it is reasonable to accept the fact that 'the earth is round' as true, because you could get into a spacecraft and prove it, it is not so easy to accept that 'I saw a ghost last night', even though I may be convinced that this is a fact.

Frame of reference

A body of knowledge which draws together facts and theories concerning some aspect of physical function or behaviour. *A primary frame of reference* includes information which originates from sources external to OT. *An applied frame of reference* is developed by occupational therapists, synthesizing material from sources both external to and within the profession. It describes the specific way in which the frame of reference is used to provide an approach to practice, usually within a speciality.

Hypothesis

A hypothesis is a 'hunch, speculation or conjecture proposed as a possible solution to a problem and requiring further investigation of its acceptability by argument or observation and experiment' (Honderich 1995). A hypothesis may be proved or disproved. It simply provides a starting point: 'I think this is what is going on ... let me see if I am right'. Therapists frequently generate hypotheses about their clients in the course of clinical reasoning.

Model (theoretical model; practice model)

A model draws together theories and knowledge from compatible but varied sources in order to integrate them and to describe or explain complex concepts. A model may offer a simplified explanation or structure to illustrate the relationships between ideas or between theory and practice. *Metamodel* is a term used by Reed (1984) to classify OT models into two divisions: *organismic (holistic)* and *mechanistic (reductionist)*.

Paradigm

1 Accepted examples of scientific practice which include law, theory appreciation and instrumentation and which represent a radically new conceptualization of phenomena (scientific: Kuhn). *Paradigm shift* describes the point at which one accepted set of ideas is abandoned in favour of a new interpretation.

2 A pattern or template which defines a set of ideas or the principles on which something is based (general usage).

3 A consensus of the most fundamental beliefs or assumptions of a field. The occupational therapy paradigm is the field's means of defining human beings and their problems in a way which suggests and provides a rationale for a course of action to solve them (OT: Kh).

Rationale

A reasoned explanation and statement of the logical basis for action.

Taxonomy

A taxonomy is a scientific system of classification in which things are named and related to each other. In OT theory the term is usually encountered in descriptions of systems for naming types of theory or for arranging the components of human occupation in a hierarchy.

Theory

'An attempt to bind together in a systematic fashion the knowledge that one has of some particular aspect of the world or experience' (Honderich 1995). A theory promotes understanding and may predict occurrences under certain conditions or offer a logical argument or set of proofs to support that what is being said is 'fact' or 'a law'. There are different types of theory. For a discussion of theory in relation to OT refer to Miller and Walker (1993) and Reed (1984).

Theory driven

The selection of a theoretical framework to guide practice before evaluating the needs of the client, as opposed to *process driven*, when the OT process is used to name and frame the client's problem before selecting an appropriate approach.

TERMS USED IN OCCUPATIONAL THERAPY

Activity analysis Dissection of an activity into its component tasks and the evaluation of therapeutic potential and relevance to the treatment plan; investigating the objective or subjective performance components. (RH)

Activity programme A programme designed to encourage individual and/or group participation through organized events for the purpose of maintaining or improving skills, roles or interactions. (RH)

Activity synthesis Combining and adapting components of an activity with components of the environment to assess performance, enhance skills or produce a desired therapeutic outcome. (RH)

Adaptation 1 Any change in structure, form or habits of an organism to suit new environment. Those changes experienced by an individual which lead to adjustment. (WS) 2 An alteration made by a therapist to an environment or an object in order to provide therapy or to improve the client's ability to function. (RH)

Adaptation to activity Modification of features such as sequence, complexity, positioning, location, use of tools, construction of equipment, to meet treatment objectives, or to improve performance.

Adaptation to environment An alteration made to a component of the physical or social environment in order to provide therapy or to improve the client's ability to function or to enhance quality of life.

Adaptive behaviour The integration of skill areas with socially accepted values to accomplish occupations and tasks. (R)

Aim A brief statement of the general purpose which treatment or intervention will be planned to achieve. (RH)

Assessment The process of collecting information, including subjective and objective data which are relevant to the preparation of an intervention plan. (R)

Client The individual who seeks the services of the therapist.

Clinical governance A framework through which National Health Service organizations in the UK are accountable for continuously improving the quality of their service through initiatives such as the use of evidence-based practice, standards, clinical audit and clinical guidelines.

Competence Skilled and adequately successful completion of a piece of performance, task or activity. The performance should be effective within defined parameters, in specified contexts, and transferred adaptively to related settings.
Professional competence involves the performance of a range of *competencies* and skills to a defined standard, within the limits of accepted boundaries and codes of conduct.

Core skills (competencies; processes) Includes therapeutic use of self, assessment, environmental and adaptation, occupational analysis and adaptation.
Basic components of professional practice which remain relatively constant although adapted by the use of frames of reference, models and approaches. (RH)

Diversional activities Those designed to alleviate boredom and to provide an enjoyable interest, without specific therapeutic intent. (RH)

Empowerment Personal and social processes that transform visible and invisible relationships so that power is shared more equally. (Townsend 1997)

Enabling Facilitating processes through which individuals or groups have the means and opportunity to be involved in solving their own problems. (Townsend 1997)
Action by an occupational therapist to assist an individual to perform occupations more easily.

Environmental adaptation Changing the physical or social features of an environment to enhance performance, promote or restrict a behaviour, or provide therapy. (RH)

Environmental analysis Observation of features in the physical or social environment and interpretation of their significance for client performance or therapy.

Facilitation 1 *Of groups:* Helpful, non-directive leadership style. (RH)
2 *Of neurodevelopmental techniques:* Specific treatment which promotes sensorimotor integration and the recovery or development of normal patterns of movement. (RH)

Functional ability (function/functional) The skill to perform activities in a normal or accepted manner. (R) Having the ability to perform competently the roles, relationships and occupations required in the course of daily life. (RH)

Goal A concise statement of a defined outcome to be attained at a particular stage in an intervention. Goals may be short term or long term.

Grading Measurable increasing or decreasing of activity, graded by length of time, size, degree of strength required or amount of energy expended. (R)

Interpersonal *Of skills:* Those which are used for interactions between people. The level, quality and/or degree of dyadic and group interaction skills. (WS)

Intervention The process of effecting change in occupational performance using meaningful occupation. (Townsend 1997) Any action taken by the therapist on behalf of the client.

Intrapersonal *Of skills:* Those which operate within the mind and emotions of the individual. (RH) The level, quality and/or degree of self-identity, self-concept and coping skills. (WS)

Medium *(pl. Media)* (modality) A therapeutic activity or agent. An agency or activity through which something is accomplished. An intervening substance through which something is transmitted or carried on. In OT, an activity or task having therapeutic potential. (R)

Objective A precise statement of the purpose, process and outcome of therapy. (RH)

Occupational therapy The treatment of physical and psychiatric conditions through specific selected activities in order to help people to reach their maximum level of function in all aspects of daily life. (WFOT) The restoration or maintenance of optimal functional independence and life satisfaction through the analysis and use of selected occupations that enable the individual to develop the adaptive skills required to support his life roles. (Cr) The use of purposeful activity with individuals who are limited by physical illness or injury, psychosocial dysfunction, developmental or learning disabilities, poverty and cultural differences, or the ageing process in order to maximize independence, prevent disability and maintain health. (AOTA)

The prescription of occupations, interactions and environmental adaptations to enable the individual to regain, develop or retain the occupational skills and roles required to maintain personal well-being and to achieve meaningful personal goals and relationships appropriate to the relevant social and cultural setting. (RH)

Occupational therapy process The sytematic form of enquiry and action used to structure intervention (obtaining information, goal setting, implementation, evaluation and review).

Outcome An agreed, predetermined, recorded, clearly defined expected result of intervention.

Outcome measure A tool which provides a means of quantifying the degree to which an outcome has been achieved.

Performance skills Skills required for successful performance of the roles that are assumed by individuals in their lives. (WS)

Personal causation Self-perception of effectiveness within the environment. (Kh)
The individual's capacity to initiate action with the intent to affect the environment. (Cr)

Problem An issue in the life of the client which prompts referral for occupational therapy. *Problem naming* is the process of identifying and recording problems which may require action. *Problem framing* is an interpretive, analytical exercise which leads to understanding of the nature of the problem in a specific context. *Problem solving* is the analytical cognitive process whereby action is selected and/or a solution to the problem is found.

Quality of life Choosing and participating in occupations that foster hope, generate motivation, offer meaning and satisfaction, and promote well-being (adapted from Townsend 1997). Life which consists of more than mundane physical existence.

Role A social or occupational identity which directs the individual's social, cultural and occupational behaviour and relationships.
Individuals typically require the capacity to carry out a variety of roles at any point in life. (RH)

Skill A specific ability or integrated set of abilities (e.g. motor, sensory, cognitive or perceptual) learnt and practised to a standard required for the effective performance of a task or subtask. (RH)

Skill analysis Analysis of a skill to identify the components required for its performance.

Techniques The body of specialized procedures and methods used in treatment. (RH)

Therapeutic alliance A style of relationship between therapist and client in which both pool knowledge and experience to address the client's needs and priorities.

Therapeutic relationship The special professional relationship which develops between client and therapist through which the therapist seeks to promote the interests and well-being of the client.

Therapy Treatment aimed at improving a health condition or providing rehabilitation following an illness or injury.

GENERAL GLOSSARY

Autonomy Personal freedom; freedom of the will. (COD)
The ability to act or perform according to one's own volition or direction. (R)
Quality of being self-governing and self-determining. (WS)

Behaviour Those activities of an organism that can be observed by another organism (or by instrumentation). Included within behaviour are verbal reports made about subjective, conscious experiences. (At)

Behaviourism Study of human actions by analysis into stimulus and response. (COD)
A branch of psychology which attempts to discover the laws that describe behaviour by relying exclusively on observable data. (Lov)

Cognition An individual's thoughts, knowledge, interpretations, understanding or ideas. (At)

Cognitive processes Mental processes of perception, memory and information processing by which the individual acquires information, makes plans and solves problems. (At)

Countertransference Conscious or unconscious responses of therapist to the patient determined by the therapist's need; transferred feelings, not necessarily relevant to the real situation. (WS)

Defence mechanism Unconscious intrapsychic process, e.g. denial, introjection, projection, rationalization. (WS)

Development The progressive and continuous change in shape, function and integration of the body from birth to death. (R)

Divergent thinking A cognitive operation in which the subject thinks in different directions. The quality of divergent thought is judged in terms of the quantity, variety and originality of the ideas produced. (Lov)

Dyadic interaction *Of skills:* Abilities in relationships to peers, subordinates and authority figures; demonstrating trust, respect and warmth; perceiving and responding to needs and feelings of others; engaging in and sustaining interdependent relationships; communicating feelings. (R)

Eclectic Borrowing freely from various sources. (COD)

Ecology (human) Study of interaction of persons with their environment. (COD)

Ethnography *In research:* A descriptive qualitative study often of an individual or situation, usually written from the perspective of the participant(s) in the first person (Polgar)

Ethnomethodology A qualitative approach to research which involves the study of social processes associated with ways in which people perceive, describe and explain the world. (Polgar)

Experiential learning A view that all learning is best gained by direct experience, which must be meaningful to the learner. (RH)

Feedback Modification or control of a process or system by its results and effects especially by difference between desired and actual result. (COD)
Information about the consequences of the actions taken by a person performing a skill. (Lov)

Gestalt psychology A system of psychological theory concerned primarily with perception that emphasizes pattern, organization, wholes and field properties. (At)

Habilitation The encouragement and stimulation of the development and acquisition of skills and functions not previously attained. (R)

Heuristic Quality that encourages further discovery or investigation. (WS)
In problem solving, a strategy that can be applied to a variety of problems that usually, but not always, provides a correct solution. (At)

Illuminative study One which recounts subjective personal experience with a view to providing insights into causes, processes and the effectiveness of procedures. (RH)

Information processing *In cognitive psychology:* The mental processes required to store, retrieve and make use of information. Models which explain or describe this process. (RH)

Input Information entering a system from the environment. (RH)

Kinesiology The study of human movement. (RH)

Modelling Setting an example for imitation (usually, of social behaviour). (RH)

Naturalistic method Techniques of research conducted in normal environments without artificial controls. (RH)

Object relations The ability of the person to invest feelings and emotions in other persons or objects. (R)

Ontogenesis Origin and development of an individual. (COD)

Ontogeny Development of an individual over the passage of time. (RH)

Open systems theory Living organisms are dynamic, self-organizing entities, exhibiting ongoing interaction with their environments. (Kh95)

Organismic A view of reality which emphasizes the subjective, interactive and holistic nature of human experience. (see Holistic; Phenomenological) (RH)

Output The product of the processes of a system. (RH)
Action of the system which produces a change in the environment; mental, physical and social aspects of occupation. (Kh)

Perception Mental process by which intellectual, sensory and emotional data are organized meaningfully; the process of conscious recognition and interpretation of sensory stimuli. (WS)

Physiology Science of functions and phenomena of living organisms and their parts. (COD)

Problem oriented medical records (POMR) A system for recording problems affecting a patient and planning and organizing action to resolve these. (RH)

Problem solving A set of cognitive strategies used to resolve difficulties. (RH)

Profession An occupation characterized by a defined body of knowledge and expertise, whose practitioners espouse a code of ethics and responsible conduct in relation to their clients. (RH)

Proprioception Appreciation of position, balance and changes in equilibrium of a body part during movement as a result of stimulus to receptors within body tissue such as muscle, tendons and joints. (WS)

Psychoanalysis A therapeutic system for the treatment of mental disorder based on the principles of analytical psychology, aimed at investigating interaction of conscious and unconscious elements in the mind and bringing the latter into consciousness. (RH)

Psychology Science of the nature, functions and phenomena of the human mind. (COD)

Psychotherapy Treatment of personality maladjustment or mental disorders by psychological means, usually, but not exclusively, through personal consultation. (At)

Qualitative methods An approach to research that emphasizes the non-numerical and interpretive analysis of social phenomena. (Polgar)

Quality assurance Activities and programmes intended to ensure the quality of care in a defined medical setting or programme. (R)

Quantitative methods An approach to research that emphasizes the collection of numerical data and the statistical analysis of hypotheses proposed by the researcher. (Polgar)

Rehabilitation Restoration to a disabled individual of maximum independence commensurate with his limitations by developing his residual capacities. (WS) The combined and coordinated use of medical, social, educational and vocational measures for training or retraining the individual to the highest possible level of functional ability. (WHO)

Rehabilitative services Those activities and procedures designed to assist a physically or mentally disabled individual to achieve or maintain the highest attainable level of function through an evaluation and treatment programme providing, under physician direction, one or a combination of medical, paramedical, psychological, social and vocational services determined by the needs of the patient.

Reliability The extent to which a test or measurement is reproducible by different people or at different times. (RH)

Self-actualization The capacity of the individual to achieve a life which fulfils potentials and offers satisfaction and personal meaning. (RH)

SOAP Heading used in POMR: Subjective; Objective; Analysis; Plan. (RH)

Standardized test One that has known characteristics, especially known levels of reliability and validity. (Polgar)

Systems theory The basis for the study of the operation of systems. Systems may be described as 'hard', i.e. of a fixed, mechanical nature; or 'soft', i.e. changing, dynamic interactions between people and environments. The operation of a system is usually described in terms of input, output, throughput and feedback. (RH)

Taxonomy Principles of classification. (COD) (Especially used in botany, biology and education)

Teleological Purposeful; relating to the view that developments are due to the purpose or design that is served by them. (COD)

Temporal Of, in or denoting time. (COD)

Transference *In psychoanalysis:* Projection of feelings, thoughts or wishes on to another who has come to represent someone from the past; inappropriate feelings applied in present context. (WS)

Validity The extent to which a test measures what it is intended to measure. (Polgar)

OCCUPATIONAL THERAPY TECHNIQUES

The definitions given below provide an explanation of some of the terms used in the text which may be unfamiliar to you. These definitions are my own, unless otherwise stated. This is not intended as a comprehensive list, but as an indication of some commonly used techniques (although some are restricted to a speciality, e.g. paediatrics, learning disabilities, or to a specific frame of reference/approach).

Techniques may be practised at different levels depending on the experience and degree of specialization of the therapist. A newly qualified therapist may have an understanding of the basic principles, and competence in frequently used techniques, but at a more advanced level the practitioner will normally require additional experience and training to become proficient and may need to work under close supervision until proficiency is attained.

Activities of daily living (ADL) assessment and training
A period of objective appraisal of an individual's functional ability when performing necessary ADL, followed by a period of training or re-education in order to improve function.

Anxiety management Techniques having a cognitive and/or behavioural basis, used to help clients to monitor and control personal anxiety levels.

Assertion training Techniques which enable the individual to appreciate personal individuality and worth, to recognize personal feelings and needs and to express these in a socially acceptable manner. Training often employs group techniques and role-play.

Behaviour modification A method of psychotherapy based on learning principles, it uses techniques such as counter-conditioning, reinforcement and shaping to modify behaviour. (At) The objective is either to remove an unproductive, injurious or antisocial behaviour or to promote positive behaviour.

Behavioural rehearsal A cognitive technique in which the client acts out and practises behaviours which are found to be difficult or stressful before attempting them in reality, and develops solutions to problems.

Biofeedback Technique in which the client is made aware of unconscious or involuntary physiological processes and learns to control them. (WS)

Chaining Technique of teaching behaviour patterns by giving reinforcement for individual components of a behaviour which may be learnt separately and then linked to form a whole. *Backward chaining* is a form of errorless learning in which a task or behaviour is taught by commencing at the point of completion and working backwards to the start.

Cognitive behaviour therapy A psychotherapy approach that emphasizes the influence of a person's beliefs, thoughts and self-statements on behaviour. Combines behaviour therapy methods with those designed to change the way the individual thinks about self and events. (At)

Compensatory techniques Those used to compensate for physical or cognitive deficit in performance, e.g. provision of adaptive equipment or environment or teaching new methods of performing tasks.

Counselling The use of client-centred techniques to enable the client to identify problems, feelings or conflicts and to reach solutions or decisions.

Desensitization Use of progressive exposure of the patient in a safe environment to a stimulus which provokes acute anxiety or other negative reaction until the point is reached where the patient can tolerate the stimulus without becoming dysfunctional.

Energy conservation Techniques including time management, time and motion study, problem solving and environmental planning enabling a patient to make maximum functional use of limited potential for energy expenditure.

Errorless learning Teaching techniques (cognitive/behavioural) which teach concepts or skills by presenting material or instruction in such a way that the possibility of failure by the learner is eliminated.

Functional assessment May include ADL assessment (see above) or may refer to specific observation and/or measurement of aspects of physical function (e.g. grip strength, mobility, range of movement).

Gaming The use of scenarios, tasks or problem solving exercises to provide groups of people with personal experience of group processes, decision making mechanisms, leadership styles or the effects of emotions, attitudes and preconceptions.

Gentle teaching A humanistic method of teaching people with learning disabilities whilst maintaining their human rights and enabling them to have an accepted place in society.

Guided fantasy Techniques in which a group leader, by means of words, images or music, provides stimulus for each individual to construct mental images, stories or journeys leading to insightful exploration of personal symbols, fantasies, desires, emotions or choices.

Home adaptations The design and provision of physical alterations to an individual's home in order to promote independent living.

Homework A term used in some cognitive techniques where a patient is given tasks to do at home usually involving a record of results and personal reactions during and after the process.

Industrial therapy Use of industrial work processes, frequently packing, assembly work or clerical work, in a simulation of a realistic work environment, with nominal pay, to assess, promote or retrain work skills.

Interviewing Techniques include formal, informal, structured and unstructured methods; interviews may be used to obtain information or to negotiate aims and objectives or to evaluate courses of action.

Joint protection Instructing patients in ways of managing personal, domestic or work activities in a manner which reduces or eliminates potentially damaging stresses on vulnerable joints. Particularly used in the management of arthritic conditions.

Lifestyle planning Techniques which enable an individual to attain a balance between the occupational elements in his/her life (work, leisure, self-care, rest) in order to reduce stress, improve quality of life, develop potentials and attain relevant personal goals.

Milieu therapy A psychotherapeutic term meaning the modification of a physical and social environment such as that provided by a therapeutic community for treatment purposes.

Mobility training Instruction of a patient in the use of mobility equipment and wheelchairs.

Neurodevelopmental techniques Techniques used in the treatment of sensorimotor disorders which are based on the use of techniques such as reflex inhibition, positioning, and sensory stimulation (e.g. Bobath, Rood, PNF). (RH)

Orthotics Assessment for, design of and production and fitting of orthoses (splints) for functional or supportive purposes, often for the upper limb.

Pacing Techniques which enable the individual to perform activities or tasks in a preplanned manner, sticking to measurable personal targets, involving use of task analysis, timed activity, rest periods, alternating types of movement, in order to maximize effective performance and minimize undesirable consequences such as pain, stress on joints or fatigue.

Perceptual training Techniques designed to train or re-educate perceptual functions such as discriminations of size, form, colour, literality, by repeated practice.

Portage A developmentally based programme constructed by a therapist enabling a parent of a handicapped child to work with the child at home, using play and care activities to achieve defined goals.

Projective techniques The use of creative media, especially art, music, modelling, writing, in a manner which encourages personal interpretations of the material and facilitates exploration of personal experiences, symbols and feelings.

Prosthetic training Techniques of instructing patients in the use of upper and lower limb prostheses following amputation.

Psychodrama The use of dramatic techniques, e.g. role play, improvisation, mime, to construct or reconstruct scenarios of significance to the participants or to engage them in experiences which will enable them to explore life themes, emotions, thoughts, reactions, relationships or defensive and coping mechanisms.

Reality orientation Used with dementing or brain damaged individuals to cue them into awareness of current time, place, persons and current circumstances. Can involve '24 hour' and 'classroom' techniques.

Relaxation Various methods involving techniques of voluntary physical or mental control designed to produce physical and mental relaxation and relieve the effects of stress or anxiety.

Reminiscence therapy (nostalgia therapy) Techniques used with dementing individuals or very elderly people in which objects from the past – photos, music, clothes, objects – are used as triggers for discussion and reflection and the sharing or validation of personal experiences and memories.

Retirement planning Techniques which enable people who have/are about to retire from work to develop a balanced and fulfilling repertoire of occupations and interests, and to maintain a healthy lifestyle.

Role-play Use of dramatic techniques and improvisation to enable patients to act out roles or situations which they wish to explore, either to gain insight into difficulties or to improve coping skills.

Room management techniques A means of providing individual attention to members of a large group for short periods, making best use of available staff and their skills, and the possibly limited attention span of participants. Typically one person acts as 'room manager' coordinating therapy, whilst another looks after physical care needs or disturbances, and one or more others spend a few minutes with each group member in turn, working for a predetermined objective.

Sensory re-education Usually carried out to restore sensitivity and discrimination of touch in the hand following peripheral nerve injury; the patient is trained to recognize a variety of progressively finer and more similar textures by touch alone.

Social modelling Shaping behaviour or attitudes by enabling the learner to observe others performing competently and gaining suitable rewards or approval for such performance.

Social skills training Educational programmes designed to improve skills of interaction and acceptable social behaviour. May use social modelling, role-play and behavioural rehearsal.

Stress management A variety of cognitive and behavioural techniques used to enable the individual to recognize signs of personal stress and to adopt positive preventative and coping strategies to reduce this.

Token economy A form of behavioural modification in which the patient is rewarded for fulfilling a specified behavioural contract by 'tokens' which are usually tradeable for goods or privileges (a behavioural technique which is now seldom used).

Vocational (work) assessment Objective appraisal of a person's abilities to perform a previous (or future) job, which may include evaluation of the need for training or the provision of compensatory equipment or environmental adaptations.

TERMS USED TO DESCRIBE OCCUPATION AND OCCUPATIONAL PERFORMANCE (Note: unless otherwise stated the definitions are the author's)

Activity A series of linked episodes of task performance which takes place on a specific occasion during a finite period for a particular reason. An activity is composed of an integrated sequence of chained tasks; a completed activity results in a change in the previous state of objective reality or subjective experience.

Activity of daily living (ADL) A basic activity required to maintain personal health and well-being. Commonly divided into: personal activities of daily living (PADL: e.g. washing, dressing, toiletting, eating); domestic activities of daily living (DADL: those associated with running a home such as cooking, cleaning, laundry); instrumental activities of daily living (IADL: used as a synonym for DADL, but including a wider range of activities such as child care, shopping, gardening, travelling around).

Environmental demand (press) The combined effect of elements of the environment which produces expectations for specific, appropriate, occupational performance.

Fit Short for 'person-activity-environment fit': refers to the match among skills and abilities of the individual, the demands of the activity and the characteristics of the physical, social and cultural environment (American Association of Occupational Therapists Uniform Terminology 1994).

Function (functional ability) Having the ability to perform competently the roles and occupations required in the course of daily life.

Leisure Activities which are freely selected by the individual in which he or she participates during self-allocated time. Leisure activities are varied and selected on the basis of meaning, pleasure, personal fulfillment, relaxation and other attributes of significance to the individual.

Meaning In relation to activities and occupations: the individual's personal attribution of significance and value, which, when positive, prompts a desire for continued or repeated participation.

Occupation 1 The dominant activity of human beings that includes serious, productive pursuits and playful, creative and festive behaviours (Kielhofner 1992).

2 Units of activity which are named in the lexicon of the culture (Occupational science: Zemke and Clark 1996).

3 Groups of activities and tasks of everyday life, named, organized and given value and meaning by individuals and a culture; occupation is everything people do to occupy themselves, including looking after themselves (self-care), enjoying life (leisure), and contributing to the economic fabric of their communities (productivity) (Canadian Occupational Performance Model: Townsend 1997).

4 A form of human endeavour which provides longitudinal organization of time and effort in a person's life.

5 A generic term for all productive human performance and behaviours: the focus of occupational therapy.

Occupational alienation A sense that one's occupations are meaningless and unfulfilling, typically associated with feelings of powerlessness to alter the situation.

Occupational behaviour (*syn* occupational performance) All actions related to engagement in occupations.

Occupational competence The ability to perform needed occupations adequately, consistently and effectively, to a required standard.

Occupational deprivation Having few occupations and/or being deprived of the opportunity to particpate in the repertoire of occupations which would normally be expected at a certain age, within a particular culture.

Occupational dysfunction A temporary or chronic inability to engage in the repertoire of roles, relationships and occupations required in the course of daily life.

Occupational identity The perceptions which an individual has of himself as an 'occupational being'; the names of occupations for which he feels ownership. Occupational identity contributes to a sense of personal identity and provides meaning to daily activities.

Occupational imbalance A lack of variety in occupation; an undue focus on one occupation to the exclusion of others.

Occupational ontogenesis The development of an individual's occupations over time.

Occupational performance The result of a dynamic, interwoven relationship between persons, environment and occupation over a person's lifespan. The ability to choose, organize and satisfactorily perform meaningful occupations that are culturally defined and age-appropriate for looking after oneself, enjoying life and contributing to the social and economic fabric of a community (Canadian Occupational Performance Model: Townsend 1997).

Occupational science An interdisciplinary academic discipline studying occupation, its origins, scope, meaning and structure.

Performance Engagement in a task or activity.

Performance areas Classifications of occupations. In the American Association of Occupational Therapists' Uniform Terminology (1994) these are designated as: activities of daily living (ADL); work and productive activities, play or leisure activities.

Role identity The roles which a person has which contribute to a sense of selfhood and place the individual in relationships with others.

Task A self-contained stage in an activity or a definable piece of performance with a completed purpose or product.

Work Work is notoriously hard to define briefly. The traditional view is that it is paid employment which provides an occupational title and role. Work has a product or result of value to society or the individual, but typically is an aspect of a division of labour which enables the individual to survive as a member of society and promotes the survival of the society as a whole. As used in OT it means the range of productive activities and tasks which the individual feels obliged to perform and to which time is allocated as a priority, because it is necessary for his own benefit or that of others.

TERMINOLOGY USED TO DEFINE DISABILITY

World Health Organization definitions

The following definitions have now been superseded, but are included as they may still be used and encountered in the literature.

Disability Loss of the ability to perform in the range considered normal for a human being.

Handicap The disadvantage or restriction of activity caused by a disability.

Impairment Damage to, loss of or pathology affecting a body organ or system or abnormality affecting psychological or physiological structure or function.

International classification of functioning and disability ICIDH-2 Beta 2 Draft (1999)

Note: this taxonomy is subject to development. At the time of writing a final version is expected in 2001. The text below is extracted from the 1999 version (www.who.int/icidh).

ICIDH-2 provides a description of situations with regard to human functioning and disability and serves as a framework to organize information according to three dimensions:

1 Body level – body functions and structure
2 Individual level – activities
3 Society level – participation

Definitions

Activity The performance of a task by an individual.

Activity limitations Difficulties an individual may have in the performance of activities.

Body function The physiological or psychological functions of body systems.

Body structures Anatomical parts of the body such as organs, limbs and their components.

Contextual factors Environmental factors (external influences on functioning) and personal factors (internal influences on functioning), together with features of the physical, social and attitudinal world and the attributes of the person.

Health condition A disorder or disease affecting the individual.

Impairments Problems in bodily function or structure such as significant deviation or loss.

Participation An individual's involvement in life situations in relation to health conditions, body functions and structure, activities and contextual factors.

Participation restrictions Problems an individual may have in the manner or extent of involvement in life situations.

RECOMMENDED READING

This appendix presents selected references mentioned in the text and additional books and articles which provide background reading for topics. The material is listed under topic headings in approximately the order in which the subjects are dealt with in the book. In some cases a short synopsis is provided.

Other references mentioned in the text can be found listed alphabetically at the end of this appendix.

SECTION 1: PHILOSOPHICAL AND THEORETICAL ASPECTS OF OCCUPATIONAL THERAPY

NATURE OF THEORY IN OT

Christiansen C 1994 Classification and study in occupation: a review and discussion of taxonomies. Journal of Occupational Science Australia 1 (3): 3–21

Miller R J 1993 What is theory and why does it matter? In: Miller R J, Walker K F (eds) Perspections on theory for the parctice of occupational therapy. Gaithersberg, Aspen

Reed K L 1984 Models of practice in occupational therapy. Williams and Wilkins, Baltimore.

Reed K L 1998 Theories that guide practice. In: Neistadt M E, Crepeau E B (eds) Willard and Spackman's Occupational therapy. Lippincott, Philadelphia

Walker K F 1993 Theory analysis. In: Miller R J, Walker K F (eds) Perspectives on theory for the practice of occupational therapy. Gaithersberg, Aspen

Young M, Quinn E 1992 Theories and practice of occupational therapy. Churchill Livingstone, Edinburgh

PHILOSOPHY AND THEORY: BACKGROUND READING

Craddock J 1996 Responses of the occupational therapy profession to the perspective of the disability movement, Part 1. British Journal of Occupational Therapy 59(1): 17–22

Craddock J 1996 Responses of the occupational therapy profession to the perspective of the disability movement,

Part 2. British Journal of Occupational Therapy 59 (2): 73–78.

Creek J (ed) 1998 Occupational therapy, new perspectives. Whurr, London

Jones D, Blair S A, Hartery T, Jones R K 1998 Sociology and occupational therapy; an integrated approach. Churchill Livingstone, Edinburgh

Honderich T (ed) 1995 The Oxford companion to philosophy. Oxford University Press, Oxford (quick reference for philosophical terms, theorists and movements)

Polifroni E C, Welch M 1999 Perspectives on the philosophy of science in nursing. Lippincott, Philadelphia (covers relevant material but from a nursing perspective)

HISTORY OF OCCUPATIONAL THERAPY

Baum C, Christiansen C 1997 The occupational therapy context: philosophy, principles, practice. In: Christiansen C, Baum C (eds) Occupational therapy: enabling function and well-being, 2nd edn. Slack, New Jersey

Miller R J, Walker K F (eds) 1993 Perspectives on theory for the practice of occupational therapy. Gaithersberg, Aspen

Patterson C F 1998 Occupational therapy and the National Health Service 1948–1998. British Journal of Occupational Therapy 61(7): 311–315

Schwartz K B 1998 The history of occupational therapy. In: Neistadt M E, Crepeau E B (eds) Willard and Spackman's Occupational therapy. Lippincott, Philadelphia

Tyldesley B 1999 The Casson Memorial Lecture: Alice Contance Owens: reflections upon a remarkable lady and a pioneer of occupational therapy in England. British Journal of Occupational Therapy 62(8): 359–366

FUTURE OF OCCUPATIONAL THERAPY

Finlayson M, Edwards J 1997 Evolving health environments and occupational therapy: definitions, descriptions and opportunities. British Journal of Occupational Therapy 60(10): 456–459

McKay E, Molineux M 2000 Occupation: reaffirming its place in our practice. British Journal of Occupational Therapy 63(5): 241–242

Nelson D L 1997 Why the profession of occupational therapy will flourish in the 21st century. The Eleanor Clark Slagle Lecture. American Journal of Occupational Therapy 51(1): 11–24

Polatajko H J 1994 Dreams, dilemmas and decisions for occupational therapy practice in a new millennium: A Canadian perspective. American Journal of Occupational Therapy 48: 590–594

Whiteford G 2000 Occupational deprivation: global challenge in the new millennium. British Journal of Occupational Therapy 63(5): 200–204

Yerxa E J 1994 Dreams, dilemmas and decisions for occupational therapy practice in a new millennium: An American perspective. American Journal of Occupational Therapy 48: 586–589

EFFECTIVENESS AND STANDARDS

Alsop A 1997 Evidence-based practice and continuing professional development. British Journal of Occupational Therapy 60(11): 503–508

Bury T, Mead J 1998 Evidence-based health care. A practical guide for therapists. Butterworth Heinemann, Oxford

Carr P 1999 A bibliography for clinical audit and evaluation of practice. British Journal of Occupational Therapy 62 (6): 262

COT 1997 Code of ethics and professional conduct for occupational therapists. British Journal of Occupational Therapy 60(1): 33–37

COT 1999 Position Statement on clinical governance. British Journal of Occupational Therapy 62(6): 261–262

Moyers P A 1999 The guide to occupational therapy practice. American Journal of Occupational Therapy 53(3): 247–322

Sealey C 1999 Clinical governance: An information guide for occupational therapists. British Journal of Occupational Therapy 62(6): 263–268

SECTION 2: MODELS OF PRACTICE IN OCCUPATIONAL THERAPY

To avoid repeated referencing, a selection of the currently available text books on occupational therapy is listed below, together with a brief note of relevant content.

These books vary in detail and approaches and it may well be necessary to refer to several in order to get a real overview of a topic. In addition the reader is recommended to delve into the additional references given in the textbooks, especially recent ones, and to study professional journals.

MODELS OF PRACTICE

Bruce M A, Borg B 1993 Psychosocial occupational therapy, frames of reference for intervention, 2nd edn. Slack, New Jersey

(Describes behavioural, developmental, cognitive behavioural, movement centred and holistic frames of reference, and the model of human occupation and cognitive disabilities model.)

Kielhofner G 1992 Conceptual foundations of occupational therapy. F A Davis, Philadelphia

(Kielhofner provides a review of the biomechanical model, cognitive-perceptual model, motor control (neurodevelopmental) model, sensory integration model (Ayres; children) and spatiotemporal adaptation model (children); group work model; model of human occupation.)

Miller R J, Walker K F 1993 Perspectives on theory for the practice of occupational therapy. Gaithersberg, Aspen

(This book takes a retrospective look at some key American theorists giving a biographical sketch and summary and critique of his or her main theoretical concepts.)

OCCUPATIONAL THERAPY THEORY AND PRACTICE

General texts

Christiansen C, Baum C (eds) 1997 Occupational therapy enabling function and well-being, 2nd edn. Slack, New Jersey

Neistadt M E, Crepeau E B 1998 Willard and Spackman's Occupational therapy, 9th edn. Lippincott, Philadelphia

Occupational therapy for physical dysfunction

Pedretti L W, Zoltan B 1996 Occupational therapy, practice skills for physical dysfunction, 4th edn. Mosby, St Louis

Trombley C A (ed) 1995 Occupational therapy for physical dysfunction, 4th edn. Williams and Wilkins, Baltimore

Turner A, Foster M, Johnson S E (eds) 1996 Occupational therapy and physical dysfunction, principles, skills and practice, 4th edn. Churchill Livingstone, Edinburgh

Occupational therapy for psychosocial dysfunction

Creek J (ed) 1997 Occupational therapy and mental health, 2nd edn. Churchill Livingstone, Edinburgh

Finlay L 1988 Occupational therapy practice in psychiatry. Croom Helm, London

Hemphill-Pearson B J 1999 Assessments in occupational therapy in mental health, an integrative approach. Slack, New Jersey

Hume C, Pullen I 1994 Rehabilitation for mental health problems: an introductory handbook, 2nd edn. Churchill Livingstone, Edinburgh

Mosey A C 1996 (reprinted) Psychosocial components of occupational therapy. Raven Press, New York

Willson M 1987 Occupational therapy in long-term psychiatry, 2nd edn. Churchill Livingstone, Edinburgh

Willson M (ed) 1996 Occupational therapy in short-term psychiatry, 3rd edn. Churchill Livingstone, Edinburgh

REFERENCES FOR SPECIFIC PHYSICAL APPROACHES

Biomechanical approaches

Chaffin D B, Andersson G B J 1991 Occupational biomechanics. Wiley, Chichester

Galley P M, Forster A L 1996 Human movement, 3rd edn. Churchill Livingstone, Edinburgh

Norkin C C, Levangie P K 1992 Joint structure and function. F A Davis, Philadelphia

Norkin C C, White D J 1985 Measurement of joint motion, a guide to goniometry. F A Davis, Philadelphia

Tyldesly B, Grieve J I 1996 Muscles, nerves and movement; kinesiology in daily living, 2nd edn. Blackwell, Oxford

Neurodevelopmental approaches

Bobath B 1990 Adult hemiplegia; evaluation and treatment. William Heinemann, London

Carr J, Shepherd R 1998 Neurological rehabilitation: optimizing motor performance. Butterworth Heinemann, Oxford

Dunn W 1997 Implementing neuroscience principles to support habilitation and recovery. In: Christiansen C, Baum C (eds) Occupational therapy enabling function and well-being, 2nd edn. Slack, New Jersey

Fisher M 1995 Stroke therapy. Butterworth Heinemann, Boston

Giles M G, Wilson C J 1993 Brain injury rehabilitation: a neurofunctional approach. Chapman and Hall, Sussex

Giuffrida C G 1998 Motor control theories and models: emerging occupational performance treatment principles and assumptions. In: Neistadt M E, Crepeau E B (eds) Willard and Spackman's Occupational therapy, 9th edn. Lippincott, Philadelphia

Jarus T 1994 Motor learning and occupational therapy: the organization of practice. American Journal of Occupational Therapy 48: 810–816

Macdonald J 1990 The international course on conductive education at the Peto Andras State Institue for Conductive Education Budapest. British Journal of Occupational Therapy 53(7): 295–300

Mathowitz V, Haugen J B 1995 Evaluation of motor behaviour, traditional and contemporary views. In: Trombley C A (ed) Occupational therapy for physical dysfunction, 4th edn. Williams and Wilkins, Baltimore

Poole J L 1991 Application of motor learning principles in occupational therapy. American Journal of Occupational Therapy 45: 531–537

Poole J L 1997 Movement related problems. In: Christiansen C, Baum C (eds) Occupational therapy, enabling function and well-being, 2nd edn. Slack, New Jersey

Pulaski K H 1998 Adult neurological dysfunction. In: Neistadt M E. Crepeau E B (eds) Willard and Spackman's Occupational therapy, 9th edn. Lippincott, Philadelphia

The Intercollegiate Working Party for Stroke, Clinical Effectiveness Evaluation Unit of the Royal College of Physicians (RCP) 2000 National Clinical Guidelines for Stroke. RCP Publications, London

United States Department of Health and Human Services 1995 Clinical practice guidelines, post stroke rehabilitation. AHCPR, Rockville, MD

Woollacott M, Shumway-Cook A 1995 Motor control: theory and practical applications. Williams and Wilkins, Baltimore

Cognitive perceptual approaches

Kielhofner G 1992 Conceptual foundations of occupational therapy. Ch 8: the cognitive perceptual model. F A Davis, Philadelphia

Riddoch M J, Humphreys G W (eds) 1994 Cognitive neuropsychology and cognitive rehabilitation. Lawrence Erlbaum Associates, East Sussex

Toglia J P 1998 Cognitive-perceptual retraining and rehabilitation. In: Neistadt M E, Crepeau E B (eds) Willard and Spackman's Occupational therapy, 9th edn. Lippincott, Philadelphia

Zoltan B, Seive E, Frieshtat B 1986 Perceptual and cognitive dysfunction in the adult stroke patient, 2nd edn. Slack, New Jersey

(see also, cognitive approaches; textbooks on physical dysfunction)

APPLIED FRAMES OF REFERENCE WHICH FOCUS ON PSYCHOSOCIAL DYSFUNCTION

Behavioural modification

Grant L, Evans A 1994 Principles of behavioural analysis. Harper Collins, London

McBrien J, Felce D 1992 Working with people who have severe learning difficulties and challenging behaviour. BIMH Publications, Clevedon

Sundel S S, Sundel M 1993 Behaviour modification in the human services, 3rd edn. Sage, London (see also cognitive behavioural approaches)

Cognitive approaches

(Related to cognition and memory)

Birnboim S 1995 A metacognitive approach to cognitive rehabilitation. British Journal of Occupational Therapy 58 (2): 61–64

Duchek J M, Abreu B C 1997 Meeting the challenge of cognitive disabilities. In: Christiansen C, Baum C (eds) Occupational therapy, enabling function and well-being, 2nd edn. Slack, New Jersey

Katz N (ed) 1992 Cognitive rehabilitation models for intervention in occupational therapy. Andover Medical, Boston

McBain K, Renton L B M 1997 Computer-assisted cognitive rehabilitation and occupational therapy. British Journal of Occupational Therapy 60(5): 199–204

Riddoch M J, Humphreys G W (eds) 1994 Cognitive neurophsychology and cognitive rehabilitation. Lawrence Erlbaum Associates, East Sussex

Toglia J M 1998 The multicontext treatment approach. In: Neistadt M E, Crepeau E B (eds) Willard and Spackman's Occupational therapy, 9th edn. Lippincott, Philadelphia

Cognitive behavioural approaches

Beck A T, Freeman A 1990 Cognitive therapy for personality disorders. Guilford Press, New York

Blackburn I, Davidson K 1990 Cognitive therapy for depression and anxiety. Blackwell Scientific, Oxford

Freeman A, Simon K, Arkowitz H, Beuther L (eds) 1989 Comprehensive handbook of cognitive therapy. Plenum, New York

Hawton K, Kirk J, Clerk D, Sallovskis P 1989 Cognitive behaviour therapy for psychiatric problems, a practical guide. Oxford University Press, Oxford

Analytical approaches

(Refer to the textbooks on OT for psychosocial disorders previously listed.)

Group work approaches

Borg B, Bruce M A 1997 Occupational therapy stories: psychosocial interaction in practice. Slack, New Jersey

Brandes D, Phillips H 1990 (reprinted) Gamesters handbook. Stanley Thornes, Cheltenham

Cole M B 1998 Group dynamics in occupational therapy: the theoretical basis and practical application of group treatment, 2nd edn. Slack, New Jersey

Finlay L 1993 Groupwork in occupational therapy. Chapman and Hall, London

Finlay L 1997 The practice of psychosocial occupational therapy, 2nd edn. Stanley Thornes, Cheltenham

Howe M C, Shwartzberg S L 1986 A functional approach to groupwork in occupational therapy. Lippincott, Philadelphia

Shwartzberg S L 1998 Group process. In: Neistadt M E, Crepeau E B (eds) Willard and Spackman's Occupational therapy, 9th edn. Lippincott, Philadelphia

Wondrake R 1998 Interpersonal skills for nurses and health care professionals. Blackwell Science, Oxford

Client-centred approaches

Blackwell B (ed) 1997 Treatment compliance and the therapeutic alliance. Overseas Publishers Association, Amsterdam

Eagan G E 1994 The skilled helper. A problem-management approach to helping, 5th edn. Wadsworth, Belmont A

Ferring V G, Law M, Clark J 1997 An occupational performance model: fostering client and therapist alliances. Canadian Journal of Occupational Therapy 64(1): 7–15

Hemphill-Pearson B J, Hunter M 1997 Holism in mental health practice. Occupational Therapy in Mental Health 13(2): 35–49

Law M 1998 Client-centred occupational therapy. Slack, New Jersey

Pelonquin S 1998 The therapeutic relationship. In: Neistadt M E, Crepeau E B (eds) Willard and Spackman's occupational therapy, 9th edn. Lippincott, Philadelphia

Rogers C 1984 Client-centred therapy: its current practice, implications and theory. Houghton Mifflin, Boston

Rogers C 1986 On becoming a person. Constable, London

Stalker K, Jones C 1998 Normalization and critical disability theory. In: Jones D, Blair S A, Hartery T, Jones R K (eds) Sociology and occupational therapy; an integrated approach. Churchill Livingstone, Edinburgh

Sumsion T (ed) 1999 Client centred practice in occupational therapy, a guide to implementation. Churchill Livingstone, Edinburgh

Webber G 1995 Gentle teaching, human occupation and social role valorisation. British Journal of Occupational Therapy 58(6): 261–263

THREE FRAMES OF REFERENCE FOR OCCUPATIONAL THERAPY A. C. MOSEY

Donohue M V 1999 Theoretical bases of Mosey's group interaction skills. Occupational Therapy International 6(1): 35–51

Miller R J, Walker K F 1993 Perspectives on theory for the practice of occupational therapy. Gaithersberg, Aspen (Ch 3 Anne Cronin Mosey)

Mosey A C 1973 Activities therapy. Raven Press, New York

Mosey A C 1981 Occupational therapy, configuration of a profession. Raven Press, New York

Mosey AC 1986 (reprinted 1996) Psychosocial components of occupational therapy. Lippincott-Raven, New York

COGNITIVE DISABILITIES MODEL C. ALLEN

Allen C K 1985 Occupational therapy for psychiatric diseases: measurement and management of cognitive disabilities. Little, Brown, Boston

Allen C K 1992 Cognitive disabilities. In: Katz N (ed) Cognitive rehabilitation: models for intervention in occupational therapy. Andover Medical Publications, Boston

Allen C K 1998 Cognitive disability frame of reference. In: Neistadt M E, Crepeau E B (eds) Willard and Spackman's Occupational therapy, 9th edn. Lippincott, Philadelphia

Allen C K, Rayner A 1996 How to start using the Allen diagnostic module: a guide to introducing Allen's theories into your practice. S&S/Worldwide, Colchester CT

Allen C K, Earhart C A, Blue T 1992 Occupational therapy treatment goals for the physically and cognitively disabled. American Occupational Therapy Association, Rockville MD

Allen C K, Earhart C A, Blue T 1993 Allen diagnostic manual. S&S/Worldwide, Colchester CT

Allen C K, Earhart C A, Blue T 1996 Allen cognitive levels documentation. S&S/Worldwide, Colchester CT

Kielhofner G 1992 Conceptual foundations of occupational therapy. Chapter 7, The cognitive disabilities model. F A Davis, Philadelphia

Miller R J, Walker K F 1993 Perspectives on theory for the practice of occupational therapy. Gaithersberg, Aspen. Ch 8

Perrin T, May H 2000 Wellbeing in dementia; an occupational approach for therapists and carers. Churchill Livingstone, Edinburgh (based on Allen's model)

Sweetingham C 1996 A critical appraisal of the cognitive disabilities model. New Zealand Journal of Occupational Therapy 47(1): 5–9

SECTION 3: PROCESSES OF CHANGE

Development

(For background to the processes of development refer to general OT textbooks.)

Matheson L N, Bohr P C 1997 Occupational competence across the lifespan. In: Christiansen C, Baum C (eds) Occupational therapy, enabling function and well-being, 2nd edn. Slack, New Jersey

Adaptation

(See references for the occupational adaptation model Schkade and Schultz.)

Rehabilitation

Goodwill C J, Chamberlain A M, Evans C (eds) 1997 Rehabilitation of physically disabled adults, 2nd edn. Croom Helm, London

(Also, refer to text books on physical occupational therapy.)

Education

Bigge M C 1992 Learning theories for teachers, 5th edn. Harper Collins, New York

Burnard P 1998 Learning human skills, 3rd edn. Butterworth Heinemann, Oxford

Gagne R M 1985 The conditions of learning and theory of instruction, 4th edn. Holt Saunders, New York

Hill W F 1999 Learning: a survey of psychological interpretations, 5th edn. McGraw Hill, Boston

Jenkins M, Brotherton C In search of a theoretical framework for practice, part 1. British Journal of Occupational Therapy 58(7): 280–284 (based on Lave's and Wenger's situated learning perspective)

Jenkins M, Brotherton C In search of a theoretical framework for practice, part 2. British Journal of Occupational Therapy 58(8): 332–336

Kiger A M 1995 Teaching for health. Churchill Livingstone, Edinburgh

McGee J J, Menolashino F J 1991 Beyond gentle teaching. Plenum Press, New York

McGill R A 1998 Motor learning: concepts and applications, 5th edn. McGraw Hill, Boston

Moore A, Hilton R, Morris J, Caladine L, Bristow H 1997 The clinical educator – role development; a self directed learning text. Churchill Livingstone, Edinburgh

Rogers C, Frieberg H J 1994 Freedom to learn, 3rd edn. Macmillan College Publishing, Ontario

SECTION 4: PERSON-ENVIRONMENT-OCCUPATIONAL PERFORMANCE MODELS

ASPECTS OF OCCUPATION

Blair S 2000 The centrality of occupation during life transitions. British Journal of Occupational Therapy 63(5): 231–237

Christiansen C 1999 The Eleanor Clark Slagle Lecture: Defining lives, occupation as identity: an essay on competence, coherence and the creation of meaning. American Journal of Occupational Therapy 53(6): 547–548

Do Rozzario L 1994 Ritual, meaning and transcendence, the role of occupation in modern life. Journal of Occupational Science Australia 1(3): 46–53

Fleming Cottrell R P (ed) 1996 Perspectives on purposeful activity, foundation and future of occupational therapy. American Occupational Therapy Association, Bethesda (collection of reprints of AJOT articles)

Gray J M 1998 Putting occupation into practice: occupation as ends; occupation as means. American Journal of Occupational Therapy 52(5): 354–364

Hasslekus B R, Rosa S A 1997 Meaning and occupation. In: Christiansen C, Baum C (eds) Occupational therapy: enabling function and well-being, 2nd edn. Slack, New Jersey

Matheson L N, Bohr P C 1997 Occupational competence across the life span. In: Christiansen C, Baum C (eds) Occupational therapy: enabling function and well-being, 2nd edn. Slack, New Jersey

Nelson D L 1996 Therapeutic occupation: a definition. American Journal of Occupational Therapy 50(10): 775–782

Reibeiro K L, Polgar J M 1999 Enabling occupational performance: optimal experiences in therapy. Canadian Journal of Occupational Therapy 66(1): 14–22

Schwammle D 1996 Occupational competence explored. Canadian Journal of Occupational Therapy 63(5): 323–330

Townsend E 1997 Occupation: potential for personal and social transformation. Journal of Occupational Science Australia 4(1): 18–26

Trombley C A 1995 Occupation: purposefulness and meaningfulness as therapeutic mechanisms (Eleanor Clark Slagle lecture). American Journal of Occupational Therapy 49: 960–972

Wilcock A A 1993 A theory of the human need for occupation. Journal of Occupational Science: Australia 1(1) 17–24

Wilcock A A 1998a An occupational perspective of health. Slack, New Jersey

Wilcock A A 1998b A theory of occupation and health. In: Creek J (ed) Occupational therapy, new perspectives. Whurr, London

Wilcock A A 1999a Reflections on doing, being and becoming. Australian Journal of Occupational Therapy 46: 1–11

Wilcock A A 1999b The Doris Sym Memorial Lecture: Developing a philosophy of occupation for health. British Journal of Occupational Therapy 62(5): 192–198

OCCUPATIONAL SCIENCE

Clark F 1993 Occupation embedded in a real life: Interweaving occupational science and occupational therapy. American Journal of Occupational Therapy 47: 1067–1078

Clark F, Parham D, Carlson ME et al 1991 Occupational science: Academic innovation in the service of occupational therapy. American Journal of Occupational Therapy 45: 300–310

Clark F, Wood W, Larson E A 1998 Occupational science: Occupational therapy's legacy for the 21st century. In: Neistadt M, Crepeau E B (eds) Willard and Spackman's Occupational therapy, 9th edn. Lippincott, Philadelphia

Illott I, Mounter C 2000 Occupational science: an impossible dream or an agenda for action? British Journal of Occupational Therapy 63(5): 238–240

Lunt A 1997 Occupational science and occupational therapy: negotiating the boundary between a discipline and a profession. Journal of Occupational Science Australia 4(2): 56–61

Mounter C, Ilott I 1997 Occupational science: a journey of discovery in the United Kingdom. Journal of Occupational Science Australia 4(2): 50–55

University of Southern California Dept. of Occupational Therapy 1989 Proposal for a PhD degree in Occupational Science (unpublished)

Yerxa E J 2000 Confessions of an occupational therapist who became a detective. British Journal of Occupational Therapy 63(5): 192–199

Yerxa E J, Clark F, Frank G et al 1990 An introduction to occupational science: a foundation for occupational therapy in the 21st century. Occupational Therapy Health Care 6: 1–17

Zemke R, Clark F 1996 Occupational science, the evolving discipline. F A Davis, Philadelphia

PEOP MODELS

Activities health: Cynkin and Robinson

Cynkin S, Robinson A M 1990 Occupational therapy and activities health: toward health through activities. Little, Brown, Boston

Model of human occupation: Reed and Sanderson

Reed K L, Sanderson S N 1992 Concepts of occupational therapy, 3rd edn. Williams and Wilkins, Baltimore

Model of human occupation: Kielhofner

Kielhofner G 1995 A model of human occupation, theory and application, 2nd edn. Williams and Wilkins, Baltimore

Kielhofner G, Barrett L 1998 The model of human occupation. In: Neistadt M, Crepeau E B (eds) Willard and Spackman's Occupational therapy, 9th edn. Lippincott, Philadelphia (Chapter 23)

Kielhofner G, Forsyth K 1997 The model of human occupation: an overview of current concepts. British Journal of Occupational Therapy 60(3): 103–110

Kyle T, Wright S 1996 Reflecting the model of human occupation in occupational therapy documentation. Australian Journal of Occupational Therapy 63(3): 192–196

Miller R J, Walker K F 1993 Perspectives on theory for the practice of occupational therapy. Ch 7 Gary Kielhofner. Gaithersberg, Aspen

Assessments (see: www.vic.edu/hsc/acad/cahp/OT/MOHO) (Published by University of Illinois, Chicago)

Baron K, Kielhofner G, Goldhammer V, Wolenski J 1998 A user's manual for the occupational self-assessment (version 1.0)

de las Heras C G, Geist R, Kielhofner G 1998 A user's guide to the volitional questionnaire (VQ) (version 3.0)

Forsyth K, Sulamy M, Simon S, Kielhofner G 1998 A user's guide to the assessment of communication and interaction skills (ACIS) (version 4.0)

Kielhofner G et al A user's manual for the occupational performance history interview (OPHI-II) (version 2.0)

Moore-Corner R A, Kielhofner G, Olson L 1998 Work environment impact scale (WEIS) (version 2.0)

Velozo C, Kielhofner G, Fisher G 1998 A user's guide to the worker role interview

Assessment of motor and process skills (AMPS)

Fisher A G 1995 Assessment of motor and process skills. Three Star Press, Fort Collins, CO

Park S, Fisher A G, Velozo C A 1994 Using the assessment of motor and process skills to compare occupational performance between clinic and home settings. American Journal of Occupational Therapy 48: 689–696

Robinson S E, Fisher A G 1996 A study to examine the relationship of the assessment of motor and process skills to other tests of cognition and function. British Journal of Occupational Therapy 59(6): 260–263

Occupational adaptation: Schkade and Schultz

Law M, Couper B A, Strong S, et al. 1997 Theoretical contexts for the practice of occupational therapy. In: Christiansen C, Baum C (eds) Occupational therapy: enabling function and well-being, 2nd edn. Slack, New Jersey.

Schkade J K, Schultz S 1992 Occupational adaptation: toward a holistic approach to contemporary practice, Part 1. American Journal of Occupational Therapy 31: 248–253

Schkade S K, Schultz S 1993 Occupational adaptation, an integrative frame of reference. In: Hopkins H, Smith H (eds) Willard and Spackman's Occupational therapy, 8th edn. Lippincott, Philadelphia

Schkade S K, Schultz S 1998 Occupational adaptation, an integrative frame of reference. In: Neistadt M, Crepeau E B (eds) Willard and Spackman's Occupational therapy, 9th edn. Lippincott, Philadelphia

Schultz S, Schkade J K 1992 Occupational adaptation: toward a holistic approach to contemporary practice, Part 2. American Journal of Occupational Therapy 46: 829–837

Schultz S, Schkade S K 1997 Adaptation. In: Christiansen C, Baum C (eds) Occupational therapy: enabling function and well-being, 2nd edn. Slack, New Jersey

Canadian occupational performance model

Bodiam C 1999 The use of the Canadian occupational performance measure for the assessment of outcome on a neurorehabilitation unit. British Journal of Occupational Therapy 62 (3): 123–125

Law M et al 1994 Canadian Occupational Performance Measure, 2nd edn. Canadian Association of Occupational Therapists, Toronto

Townsend E et al (eds) 1997 Enabling occupation: an occupational therapy perspective. Canadian Association of Occupational Therapists, Ottawa

Competent occupational performance in the environment (COPE): Hagedorn

Hagedorn R 1995 Perspectives and processes in occupational therapy. Churchill Livingstone, Edinburgh

Hagedorn R 2000 Tools for practice in occupational therapy. Churchill Livingstone, Edinburgh

REFERENCES

Allen C K 1985 Occupational therapy for psychiatric diseases: measurement and management of cognitive disabilities. Little, Brown, Boston

American Association of Occupational Therapists 1995 The philosophical base of occupational therapy. American Journal of Occupational Therapy 49(10): 1026

Arnold M E, Penn B 1990 Expert systems and occupational therapy. British Journal of Occupational Therapy 53(9): 365–368

Atkinson R L, Atkinson R G, Smith E, Benn D 1993 Introduction to psychology, 11th edn. Harcourt Brace Jovanovich, Florida

Ayres A J 1973 Sensory integration and learning disorders. Western Psychological Services, Los Angeles CA

Balóueff O 1998 Sensory integration. In: Neistadt M, Crepeau E B (eds) Willard and Spackman's Occupational therapy, 9th edn. Lippincott, Philadelphia

Bandura A 1977a Social learning theory. Prentice Hall

Bandura A 1977b Self-efficacy: towards a unifying theory of behaviour change. Psychological Review 84: 191–215

Barnitt R 1998 In: Creek J (ed) Occupational therapy: new perspectives. Whurr, London

Baron R A, Byrne D 1987 Social psychology, 5th edn. Allyn and Bacon, Massachussetts

Baron K, Kielhofner G, Goldhammer V, Wolenski J 1998 A user's manual for the occupational self-assessment (version 1.0). University of Illinois, Chicago

Beck A T, Freeman A 1990 Cognitive therapy for personality disorders. Guilford Press, New York

Birnboim S 1995 A metacognitive approach to cognitive rehabilitation. British Journal of Occupational Therapy 58(2): 61–64

Bobath B 1990 Adult hemiplegia evaluation and treatment, 3rd edn. William Heinemann Medical Books, London

Bruner J 1990 Acts of meaning. Harvard University Press, Cambridge Mass

Brunnstrom S 1970 Movement therapy in hemiplegia. Harper and Row, New York

Burke J P, De Poy E 1991 An emerging view of mastery excellence and leadership in occupational therapy practice. American Journal of Occupational Therapy 45(1): 1027–1032

Bury T, Mead J 1998 Evidence-based health care. A practical guide for therapists. Butterworth Heinemann, Oxford

CAOT 1997 Enabling occupation: an occupational therapy perspective. Canadian Association of Occupational Therapists, Ottawa

Carr J, Shepherd R, 1998 Neurological rehabilitation: optimizing motor performance. Butterworth Heinemann, Oxford

Christiansen C 1999 The Eleanor Clark Slagle Lecture: Defining lives, occupation as identity: an essay on competence, coherence and the creation of meaning. American Journal of Occupational Therapy 53(6): 547–548

Christiansen C, Baum C (eds) 1997 Occupational therapy enabling function and well-being, 2nd edn. Slack, New Jersey

Clark F, Ennevor B L, Richardson P (posthumously) 1996 A grounded theory of techniques for occupational storytelling and storymaking. In: Zemke R, Clark F (eds) Occupational science, the evolving discipline. F A Davis, Philadelphia

Clark F, Wood W, Larson E A 1998 Occupational science: Occupational therapy's legacy for the 21st century. In: Neistadt M, Crepeau E B (eds) Willard and Spackman's Occupational therapy, 9th edn. Lippincott, Philadelphia

Collins M 1998 Occupational therapy and spirituality: reflecting on quality of experience in therapeutic interventions. British Journal of Occupational Therapy 61(6): 280–284

COT 1997 Code of ethics and professional conduct for occupational therapists. British Journal of Occupational Therapy 60(1): 33–37

COT 1999 Position statement on clinical governance. British Journal of Occupational Therapy 62(6): 261–262

Craik C, Austin C, Chacksfield J, Ricards G, Schell D 1998 College of occupational therapists: Position paper on the way ahead for research, education and practice in mental health. British Journal of Occupational Therapy 61(9): 390–392

Creek J (ed) 1997 Occupational therapy and mental health, 2nd edn. Churchill Livingstone, Edinburgh

Creek J 1997 The truth is no longer out there. British Journal of Occupational Therapy 6(2): 50–52

Cynkin S, Robinson A M 1990 Occupational therapy and activities health: toward health through activities. Little, Brown, Boston

de las Heras C G, Geist R, Kielhofner G 1998 A users guide to the volitional questionnaire (VQ) (version 3.0). University of Illinois, Chicago

Department of National Health and Welfare and the CAOT 1983 Guidelines for the client-centred practice of occupational therapy. H39/33/1983e. Ottawa, Ontario

Department of National Health and Welfare and the CAOT 1986 Intervention guidelines. H39/100/1986e. Ottawa, Ontario

Department of National Health and Welfare and the CAOT 1987 Towards outcome measures in occupational therapy. H39/114/1987e. Ottawa, Ontario

Do Rozzario L 1994 Ritual, meaning and transcendence, the role of occupation in modern life. Journal of Occupational Science Australia 1(3): 46–53

Duchek J M, Abreu B C 1997 Meeting the challenge of cognitive disabilities. In: Christiansen C, Baum C (eds) Occupational therapy, enabling function and well-being, 2nd edn. Slack, New Jersey

Dunn W 1997 Implementing neuroscience principles to support habilitation and recovery. In: Christiansen C, Baum C (eds) Occupational therapy enabling function and well-being, 2nd edn. Slack, New Jersey

Fisher A G 1994 Assessment of motor and process skills. Three Star Press, Fort Collins CO

Forsyth K, Sulamy M, Simon S, Kielhofner G 1998 A user's guide to the assessment of communication and interaction skills (ACIS) (version 4.0). University of Illinois, Chicago

Giuffrida C G 1998 Motor control theories and models: emerging occupational performance treatment principles and assumptions. In: Neistadt M E, Crepeau E B (eds) Willard and Spackman's Occupational therapy, 9th edn. Lippincott, Philadelphia

Golisz K M, Toglia J P 1998 Evaluation of perception and cognition. In: Neistadt M E, Crepeau E B (eds) Willard and Spackman's Occupational therapy, 9th edn. Lippincott, Philadelphia

Gore S 1997 Management. In: Creek J (ed) Occupational therapy and mental health, 2nd edn. Churchill Livingstone, Edinburgh

Hagedorn R 1995a Perspectives and processes in occupational therapy. Churchill Livingstone, Edinburgh

Hagedorn R 1995b The first intervention: an exploratory study of clinical decison making in occupational therapy. Unpublished thesis

Hagedorn R 2000 Tools for practice in occupational therapy. Churchill Livingstone, Edinburgh

Hasslekus B R, Rosa S A 1997 Meaning and occupation. In: Christiansen C, Baum C (eds) Occupational therapy: enabling function and well-being, 2nd edn. Slack, New Jersey

Hawes D 1996 Against Postmodernism: a Marxist perspective. British Journal of Occupational Therapy 59(3): 131–132

Helfrich C, Kielhofner G 1994 Volitional narratives and the meaning of therapy. American Journal of Occupational Therapy 48: 318–326

Honderich T (ed) 1995 The Oxford companion to philosophy. Oxford University Press, Oxford

Hopkins H, Smith H (eds) 1993 Willard and Spackman's Occupational therapy, 8th edn. Lippincott, Philadelphia

Horak F B 1991 Assumptions underlying motor control for neurological rehabilitation. In: Lister M J (ed) Contemporary management of motor control problems. Proceedings of the II Step Conference, pp 11–27. Bookcrafters, Fredericksburg, VA

Hume C 1999 Spirituality: a part of total care? British Journal of Occupational Therapy 62(8): 367–370

Johnson S E 1996 Management and the occupational therapist. In: Turner A, Foster M, Johnson S (eds) Occupational therapy and physical dysfunction. Churchill Livingstone, Edinburgh

Journal of Occupational Science Australia 1994 1(3): 21 (anon)

Kaplan K, Kielhofner G 1989 Occupational case analysis interview and rating scale. Slack, New Jersey

Kielhofner G 1980a A model of human occupation, part 2. Ontogenesis from the perspective of temporal adaptation. American Journal of Occupational Therapy 34(10): 657–663

Kielhofner G 1980b A model of human occupation, part 3. Benign and vicious cycles. American Journal of Occupational Therapy 34(11): 731–737

Kielhofner G 1992 Conceptual foundations of occupational therapy. F A Davis, Philadelphia

Kielhofner G 1995 A model of human occupation, theory and application, 2nd edn. Williams and Wilkins, Baltimore

Kielhofner G, Burke JP 1980 A model of human occupation, part 1. Conceptual framework and content. American Journal of Occupational Therapy 34(9): 572–581

Kielhofner G, Burke JP, Igi H 1980 A model of human occupation, part 4. Assessment and intervention. American Journal of Occupational Therapy 34(12): 777–778

Kielhofner G et al 1998 A user's manual for the occupational, performance history interview (OPHI-II) (version 2.0). University of Illinois, Chicago

Kings Fund Centre 1988 The problem orientated medical record (POMR): guidelines for therapists. Kings Fund Centre, London

Kleinman B L, Buckley B L 1982 Some implications of a science of adaptive responses. American Journal of Occupational Therapy 36: 15–19

Knott M, Voss D 1968 Proprioceptive neuromuscular facilitation. Harper and Row, New York

Knowles M 1978 The adult learner: a neglected species. Gulf, Houston

Kortman B 1994 The eye of the beholder: models in occupational therapy. Australian Journal of Occupational Therapy 41: 115–122

Law M 1998 Client-centred occupational therapy. Slack, New Jersey

Law M, Baptist F, Carswell H et al 1994 Canadian occupational performance measure, 2nd edn. Canadian Association of Occupational Therapists, Toronto

Law M, Couper B A, Strong S et al 1997 Theoretical contexts for the practice of occupational therapy. In: Christiansen C, Baum C (eds) Occupational therapy: Enabling functional and well-being, 2nd edn. Slack, New Jersey

Levy L L 1993 Cognitive disability frame of reference. In: Willard and Spackman's Occupational therapy. Lippincott, Philadelphia,

Llorens L A 1970 Facilitating growth and development; the promise of occupational therapy. American Journal of Occupational Therapy 22: 286–288

Llorens L A 1976 Application of a developmental theory for rehabilitation and health. American Occupational Therapy Association, Rockville MD

Macdonald J 1990 The international course on conductive education at the Peto Andras State Institute for

Conductive Education Budapest. British Journal of Occupational Therapy 53(7): 295–300

Mattingly C, Fleming M H 1994 Clinical reasoning: forms of enquiry in a therapeutic practice. F A Davis, Philadelphia

McBain K, Renton L B M 1997 Computer-assisted cognitive rehabilitation and occupational therapy. British Journal of Occupational Therapy 60(5): 199–204

McColl M A, Gerein N, Valentine F 1997 Meeting the challenges of disability: models for enabling function and well-being. In: Christiansen C, Baum C (eds) Occupational therapy, enabling function and well-being, 2nd edn. Slack, New Jersey

Meyer A 1922 The philosophy of occupational therapy. American Journal of Occupational Therapy (1977) 31: 639–642

Miller R J 1993 What is theory and why does it matter? In: Miller R J, Walker K F (eds) Perspectives on theory for the practice of occupational therapy. Gaithersberg, Aspen

Miller R J, Walker K F (eds) 1993 Perspectives on theory for the practice of occupational therapy. Gaithersberg, Aspen

Moore-Corner R A, Kielhofner G, Olson L 1998 Work environment impact scale (WEIS) (version 2.0). University of Illinois, Chicago

Mosey A C 1986 (reprinted 1996) Psychosocial components of occupational therapy, Lippincott-Raven Publications, New York

Mullins L J 1993 Management and organisational behaviour, 3rd edn. Pitman, London

Neistadt M E, Crepeau E B 1998 Willard and Spackman's Occupational therapy, 9th edn. Lippincott, Philadelphia

Nelson D L 1988 Occupation: form and performance. American Journal of Occupational Therapy 42: 633–641

Nelson D L 1996 Therapeutic occupation: a definition. American Journal of Occupational Therapy 50(10): 775–782

Nelson D L 1997 Why the profession of occupational therapy will flourish in the 21st century. The Eleanor Clark Slagle Lecture. American Journal of Occupational Therapy 51(1): 11–24

Newell A 1977 On the analysis of human problem solving protocols. In: Johnson-Laird P N, Wason PC (eds) Thinking: readings in cognitive science. Cambridge University Press, Cambridge

Polatajko H J 1994 Dreams, dilemmas and decisions for occupational therapy practice in a new millenium: A Canadian perspective. American Journal of Occupational Therapy 48: 590–594

Poole J L 1997 Movement related problems. In: Christiansen C, Baum C (eds) Occupational therapy, enabling function and well-being, 2nd edn. Slack, New Jersey

Pulaski K H 1998 Adult neurological dysfunction. In: Neistadt M E, Crepeau E B (eds) Willard and Spackman's Occupational therapy, 9th edn. Lippincott, Philadelphia

Reed K L 1984 Models of practice in occupational therapy. Williams and Wilkins, Baltimore

Reed K L 1998 Theories that guide practice. In: Neistadt M E, Crepeau E B (eds) Willard and Spackman's Occupational therapy 59th (eds). Lippincott, Philadelphia

Reed K L, Sanderson S N 1980 Concepts of occupational therapy. Williams and Wilkins, Baltimore

Rogers J C, Holm M B 1991 Occupational therapy: diagnostic reasoning, a component of clinical reasoning. American Journal of Occupational Therapy 45(11): 1045–1053

Rood M 1956 Neurophysiological mechanisms utilized in the treatment of neuromuscular dysfunction. American Journal of Occupational Therapy 10: 220–225

Rose A 1999 Spirituality and palliative care: the attitudes of occupational therapists. British Journal of Occupational Therapy 62(7): 307–312

Schell B B 1998 Clinical reasoning: the basis of practice. In: Neistadt M E, Crepeau E B (eds) Willard and Spackman's Occupational therapy, 9th eds. Lippincott, Philadelphia

Schkade J K, Schultz S 1992 Occupational adaptation: toward a holistic approach to contemporary practice, Part 1. American Journal of Occupational Therapy 31: 248–253

Schkade S K, Schultz S 1998 Occupational adaptation, an integrative frame of reference. In: Neistadt M, Crepeau E B (eds) Willard and Spackman's Occupational therapy, 9th edn. Lippincott, Philadelphia

Schon D 1983 The reflective practitioner: how professionals think in action. Basic Books, USA

Schultz S, Schkade J K 1992 Occupational adaptation: toward a holistic approach to contemporary practice, Part 2. American Journal of Occupational Therapy 46: 829–837

Schultz S, Schkade S K 1997 Adaptation. In: Christiansen C, Baum C (eds) Occupational therapy: enabling function and well-being, 2nd edn. Slack, New Jersey

Schwartz K B 1998 The history of occupational therapy. In: Neistadt M E, Crepeau E B (eds) 1998 Willard and Spackman's Occupational therapy, 9th eds. Lippincott, Philadelphia

Sealey C 1999 Clinical governance: An information guide for occupational therapists. British Journal of Occupational Therapy 62(6): 263–268

Slater D Y, Cohn E S 1991 Staff development through the analysis of practice. American Journal of Occupational Therapy 45(11): 1038–1044

Sussenberger B B 1998 Socioeconomic factors and their influence on occupational performance. In: Neistadt M E, Crepeau E B (eds) Willard and Spackman's Occupational therapy, 9th eds. Lippincott, Philadelphia

The Intercollegiate Working Party for Stroke, Clinical Effectiveness Evaluation Unit of the Royal College of Physicians (RCP) 2000 National Clinical Guidelines for Stroke. RCP Publications, London

Toglia J P 1991 Generalization of treatment: a multicontext approach to cognitive perceptual impairment in the brain injured adult. American Journal of Occupational Therapy 45: 505–516

Toglia J P 1998a The multicontext treatment approach. In: Neistadt M E, Crepeau E B (eds) Willard and Spackman's Occupational therapy, 9th edn. Lippincott, Philadelphia

Toglia J P 1998b Cognitive-perceptual retraining and rehabilitation. In: Neistadt M E, Crepeau E B (eds) Willard and Spackman's Occupational therapy, 9th edn. Lippincott, Philadelphia

Tornebohm H 1991 What is worth knowing in occupational therapy? American Journal of Occupational Therapy 45: 451–454

Townsend E 1997 Occupation: potential for personal and social transformation. Journal of Occupational Science Australia 4(1): 18–26

Trombley C A (ed) 1995a Occupational therapy for physical dysfunction, 4th edn. Williams and Wilkins, Baltimore

Trombley C A 1995b Occupation: purposefulness and meaningfulness as therapeutic mechanisms. Eleanor Clark Slagle lecture. American Journal of Occupational Therapy 49: 960–972

Turner A, Foster M, Johnson S E (eds) 1996 Occupational therapy and physical dysfunction. Principles, skills and practice, 4th edn. Churchill Livingstone, Edinburgh

Tyldesley B 1999 The Casson Memorial Lecture: Alice Contance Owens: reflections upon a remarkable lady and a pioneer of occupational therapy in England. British Journal of Occupational Therapy 62(8): 359–366

United States Department of Health and Human Services 1995 Clinical practice guidelines: post stroke rehabilitation. AHCPR, Rockville, MD

Van Bruggen H 2000 A survey of models of practice taught in European Schools of Occupational Therapy. ENOCE (in preparation)

Velozo C, Kielhofner G, Fisher G 1998 A user's guide to the worker role interview. University of Illinois, Chicago

Webber G 1995 Gentle teaching, human occupation and social role valorisation. British Journal of Occupational Therapy 58(6): 261–263

Weed L L 1968 Medical records that guide and teach. New England Journal of Medicine 278: 593–599

Weed L L 1969 Medical records, medical education and patient care. Western Reserve University, Cleveland

Wilcock A A 1993 A theory of the human need for occupation. Journal of Occupational Science Australia 1(1): 17–24

Wilcock A A 1998a An occupational perspective of health. Slack New Jersey

Wilcock A A 1998b A theory of occupation and health. In: Creek J (ed) Occupational therapy, new perspectives. Whurr, London

Wilcock A A 1999a Reflections on doing, being and becoming. Australian Journal of Occupational Therapy 46: 1–11

Wilcock A A 1999b The Doris Sym Memorial Lecture: Developing a philosophy of occupation for health. British Journal of Occupational Therapy 62(5): 192–198

Wilsdon J 1996 Introduction to neurology. In: Turner A, Foster M, Johnson S (eds) Occupational therapy and physical dysfunction. Churchill Livingstone, Edinburgh

Yerxa E J 1994 Dreams, dilemmas and decisions for occupational therapy practice in a new millennium: An American perspective. American Journal of Occupational Therapy 48: 586–589

Young M, Quinn E 1992 Theories and practice of occupational therapy. Churchill Livingstone, Edinburgh

Yura H, Walsh M S 1988 The nursing process: assessing, planning, implementing, evaluating, 5th edn. Appleton and Lange, Norwalk, CT

Zemke R, Clark F (eds) Occupational science: the evolving discipline. F A Davis, Philadelphia, PA

Index

Notes: page references in *italics* are to tables and boxes; those in **bold** are to glossary definitions. Abbreviations used are: AFR = applied frame of reference; COPE = Competent Occupational Performance in the Environment; MOHO = model of human occupation; OT = occupational therapy; OTs = occupational therapists; PEOP = Person–Environment–Occupational Performance.